An Introduction to Natural Computation

Complex Adaptive Systems
John H. Holland, Christopher G. Langton, and Stewart W. Wilson, advisors

Adaption in Natural and Artificial Systems: An Introductory Analysis with Applications to Biology, Control, and Artificial Intelligence, John H. Holland

Toward a Practice of Autonomous Systems: Proceedings of the First European Conference on Artificial Life, edited by Francisco J. Varela and Paul Bourgine

Genetic Programming: On the Programming of Computers by Means of Natural Selection, John R. Koza

Genetic Programming: The Movie, John R. Koza and James P. Rice

From Animals to Animats 2: Proceedings of the Second International Conference on Simulation of Adaptive Behavior, edited by Jean-Arcady Meyer, Herbert L. Roitblat, and Stewart W. Wilson

Intelligent Behavior in Animals and Robots, David McFarland and Thomas Bösser

Advances in Genetic Programming, edited by Kenneth E. Kinnear, Jr.

Genetic Programming II: Automatic Discovery of Reusable Programs, John R. Koza

Genetic Programming II Video: The Next Generation, John R. Koza

Turtles, Termites, and Traffic Jams: Explorations in Massively Parallel Microworlds, Mitchel Resnick

From Animals to Animats 3: Proceedings of the Third International Conference on Simulation of Adaptive Behavior, edited by Dave Cliff, Philip Husbands, Jean-Arcady Meyer, and Stewart W. Wilson

Artificial Life IV: Proceedings of the Fourth International Workshop on the Synthesis and Simulation of Living Systems, edited by Rodney A. Brooks and Pattie Maes

Comparative Approaches to Cognitive Science, edited by Herbert L. Roitblat and Jean-Arcady Meyer

Artificial Life: An Overview, edited by Christopher G. Langton

Evolutionary Programming IV: Proceedings of the Fourth Annual Conference on Evolutionary Programming, edited by John R. McDonnell, Robert G. Reynolds, and David B. Fogel

An Introduction to Genetic Algorithms, Melanie Mitchell

Catching Ourselves in the Act: Situated Activity, Interactive Emergence, and Human Thought, Horst Hendriks-Jansen

Toward a Science of Consciousness: The First Tucson Discussion and Debates, edited by Stuart R. Hameroff, Alfred W. Kaszniak, and Alwyn C. Scott

Genetic Programming: Proceedings of the First Annual Conference, edited by John R. Koza, David E. Goldberg, David B. Fogel, and Rick L. Riolo

Evolutionary Programming V: Proceedings of the Fifth Annual Conference on Evolutionary Programming, edited by Lawrence J. Fogel, Peter J. Angeline, and Thomas Bäck

Elements of Artificial Neural Networks, Kishan Mehrotra, Chilukuri K. Mohan, and Sanjay Ranka

From Animals to Animats 4: Proceedings of the Fourth International Conference on Simulation of Adaptive Behavior, edited by Pattie Maes, Maja J. Mataric, Jean-Arcady Meyer, and Stewart W. Wilson

Advances in Genetic Programming, Volume 2, edited by Peter J. Angeline and Kenneth E. Kinnear, Jr.

Growing Artificial Societies: Social Science from the Bottom Up, Joshua M. Epstein and Robert Axtell

Artificial Life V: Proceedings of the Fifth International Workshop on the Synthesis and Simulation of Living Systems, edited by Christopher G. Langton and Katsunori Shimohara

An Introduction to Natural Computation, Dana H. Ballard

An Introduction to Natural Computation

Dana H. Ballard

A Bradford Book
The MIT Press
Cambridge, Massachusetts
London, England

This book was set in Palatino by Omegatype, Inc., and was printed and bound in the United States of America.

Library of Congress Cataloging-in-Publication Data
Ballard, Dana Harry.
    An introduction to natural computation / Dana H. Ballard.
      p. cm.—(Complex adaptive systems)
    Includes index.
    ISBN 0-262-02420-9 (hardcover : alk. paper)
    1. Brain—Computer simulation. I. Title. II. Series.
QP356.B345 1997
573.8′6′011363—dc21   96-44545
                                 CIP

Contents

Figures

Tables

Preface

One of the last great challenges is to understand the functioning of the human brain, and it is now clear that the brain is unlikely to be understood without recourse to computational theories. This book attempts to circumscribe the computational material that will form the underpinning of the ultimate set of brain models.

Many excellent texts, from *Introduction to the Theory of Neural Computation* by John Hertz, Anders Krogh, and Richard G. Palmer (Redwood City, CA: Addison-Wesley, 1991) to *Neural Networks for Pattern Recognition* by Christopher M. Bishop (New York: Oxford University Press, 1995), have appeared in recent years. This book differs from both of those in several ways. First, it stresses a broad spectrum of learning models, ranging from neural network learning through reinforcement learning to genetic learning. Second, it attempts to situate the various models in their appropriate neural context. Third, it attempts to make the material accessible to advanced undergraduates as well as beginning graduate students.

Writing about models of the brain before the brain has been fully understood is a delicate matter. One extreme is to make very detailed models of the neural circuitry. The danger that such models need to avoid is losing track of the task that the brain might be trying to solve. The other extreme is to have very abstract models that can represent cognitive constructs that can be readily tested. The danger that these models need to avoid is becoming so abstract that they lose track of all relationships to neurobiology. This book tries to walk a middle ground by choosing a level of discourse that stresses the computational task while at the same time staying near the neurobiology.

The overall theme of the book is that ideas from diverse areas such as neuroscience, information theory, and optimization theory have recently been extended in a way that makes them useful for describing the brain's programs. The many different sources for these ideas are acknowledged at the end of each chapter. In addition I am grateful for permission to use the many figures that illustrate particular points.

Writing any book is a monumental undertaking. I could not have done it without the inspiration of many exceptional doctoral students. The innovative work of Virginia de Sa, Jonas Karlsson, Andrew McCallum, Polly

Pook, Rajesh Rao, Justinian Rosca, Ramesh Sarukkai, Patrice Simard, and Steve Whitehead lends its sparkle to these pages.

In addition, I have benefited greatly from many discussions with my colleagues at the University of Rochester, especially Christopher Brown and Randal Nelson from the Department of Computer Science and Charlie Duffy, Mary Hayhoe, Peter Lennie, Bill Merigan, Gary Paige, Tania Pasternak, Mark Schieber, and Dave Williams through the Center for Visual Science.

The overall framework for the book has been shaped by many heated discussions by the Woods Hole Workshop on Computational Neuroscience, the brainchild of Terry Sejnowski from the Salk Institute and Joel Davis from the Office of Naval Research, and additionally by experiments made possible through the National Institutes of Health Research Resource at Rochester.

Beside trial runs at Rochester, a draft of the book has been used as a text by Hans Knutsson at Linköping University in Sweden. I am eternally thankful for the work done by Hans and his students in discovering many typographical errors.

A special thanks goes to Peg Meeker who worked with me to refine all aspects of the manuscript and guide it through its LaTeX birth. We both rave about Textures, an excellent piece of software for the Macintosh. We could not have succeeded, moreover, without the software expertise of Liudrikas Bukys.

I have been generously supported by the National Science Foundation through Howard Moraff and by the National Institutes of Health through Richard DuBois.

Last, I would like to thank Janie for our long walk together. I love you.

An Introduction to Natural Computation

1 Natural Computation

1.1 INTRODUCTION

One of the most exciting challenges of our time is to understand animal intelligence. Such a quest necessarily has as its focus a model of animal brains and most importantly a model of the operation of the human brain.

> The central tenet of modern neural science is that all behavior is a reflection of brain function. According to this view . . . what we commonly call mind is a range of functions carried out by the brain. The action of the brain underlies not only relatively simple motor behaviors such as walking, breathing and smiling, but also elaborate affective and cognitive behaviors such as feeling, learning, thinking and composing a symphony.[1]

Enormous progress has been made toward understanding the brain at many different levels, from the molecular to the biophysical. We now are zeroing in on detailed models of neurotransmitter chemistry and genetic structure. As we begin to understand the complexity of these underlying processes, a growing consensus is that *computational models*[2] will play a vital role in a complete picture of brain function, particularly in modeling more macroscopic structures that may be directly related to our conscious perceptions.

Computational models seek to characterize how the brain acquires and uses information in behavior. Interest in computational models, particularly in computational models of learning, has virtually exploded in the past decade for a number of reasons. One is the development of an array of new computational methods. Another is the continuing improvement in the speed of computers, which has made the simulation of very large systems possible. A third reason is the cross-pollination of computational models with experimental methods; brain-imaging methods are developing to the point where computational models can be directly tested. The purpose of this book is to serve as an introduction to the computational models that are spurring these new developments.

That the brain could be described by computation is itself controversial. The issue is that computation is a weak model, and, as we will see in a moment, most of the key theoretical results from computer science are about limitations. The key question, however, is, Is computation sufficient to model the brain? One view is negative, and this is articulated in Roger Penrose's critiques.[3] Penrose thinks that the extra structure of quantum physics may have additional power. This text, on the other hand, articulates a more mainstream and positive view: Computation is a weak model, but emergent evidence suggests that it may be good enough. Taking just two examples:

• A driving algorithm learns correspondences between road images and steering commands.[4] On its first tests, it drives Carnegie Mellon University's automated van ten times faster than had previously been possible.

• A game-playing algorithm learns to play world-class backgammon, having tied the world champion.[5] A key element is that it can play itself and constantly improve.

While these algorithms cannot violate the laws of computation, they do make use of a number of computational insights that break with the tenets of classical computing. These insights stem directly from the use of computational models to understand brain function, and they form the focus of this book. To highlight them, we use the title *An Introduction to Natural Computation*, borrowing a phrase coined by Whitman Richards.[6] Richards's goal was to describe the necessary inferences a biological system must make given that its computational abilities are limited. There could be no better introduction to the scope of this book:

Biological systems have available through their senses only very limited information about the external world. Yet these systems make strong assertions about the actual state of the world outside themselves. These assertions are of necessity incomplete. Clearly, a replica of an object and its qualities cannot be embodied within the brain. How can an incomplete description, encoded within neural states, be sufficient to direct the survival and successful adaptive behavior of a living system?[7]

1.2 THE BRAIN

The brain is an exquisitely beautiful structure that has evolved over millennia to perform very specific functions related to animal survival and procreation. It is a very complex structure that can be understood only by studying its features at different spatial scales.[8]

1.2.1 Subsystems

At the largest scale, the brain has specialized mechanisms for input, output, short-term memory, long-term memory, and arousal. The functions of the major subsystems are far from completely understood, but Table 1.1 will serve to orient you.

When it comes to computation, the most important parts of the brain are the cerebral hemispheres and their immediately associated structures. Each of these has a special function as shown in Figure 1.1.[9]

Table 1.1 The organization of the brain into a layered anatomical structure with increasing refinement of function culminating with the site of complex programs and memory in the cerebral hemispheres.

Component	Function
Cerebral hemispheres	The cortex, basal ganglia, hippocampus, and amygdaloid nucleus form the site of the brain's complex programs and memory
Diencephalon	Thalamus: cortical I/O; hypothalamus: regulation of autonomic, endocrine, and visceral function
Midbrain	Eye movement control; visual and auditory reflexes
Medulla oblongata	Peripheral circuitry to control autonomic functions, e.g., digestion, breathing, heart rate
Pons	Interface between cerebellum and cerebral hemispheres
Spinal cord	Peripheral circuitry to control movement of limbs and trunk; receives and processes sensory information

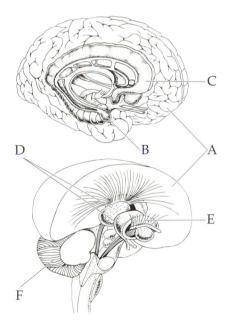

Figure 1.1 The basic function units of the human brain: (*A*) cortex: associated with long-term memory; (*B*) amygdala: associated with arousal or characterizing the importance of the current processing; (*C*) hippocampus: associated with recording working memory, that is, the variables used in the current programs; (*D*) thalamus: associated with input and output modulation; (*E*) basal ganglia: associated with the establishment of sequential programs; contains a prominent chemical reward system; (*F*) cerebellum: associated with motor "memory" or learned sensorimotor subroutines. (From Pansky and Allen, 1980; reproduced from *Review of Neuroscience,* © 1980, Macmillan, with permission of the McGraw-Hill Companies.)

• The *cortex* is the main site of the brain's permanent memory. It has the structure of a six-layered sheet of neurons and is specialized into different regions. The cortex is the most studied part of the brain, and the most studied region of cortex is that at the back of the brain, which is responsible for vision.

• The *basal ganglia* is a region in the center of the brain that plays a major role in sequential actions that are central to complex behaviors. It has elaborate chemical reward systems for rating the value of different action sequences. These are essential as a fundamental problem is estimating the value of current behaviors that are done for future rewards.

• The *hippocampus* plays a central role in the permanent recording of momentary experiences. Of the deluge of ongoing experiences in the brain, what is worth remembering? The hippocampus has mechanisms for registering current experiences until they can be stored more permanently. For people who have injured their hippocampus, time stops at the point of injury; they can participate in conversations, behaviors, and the like but do not remember them.

• The *cerebellum* plays the major role in the memory for complicated sensorimotor experiences associated with actions. Catching a baseball in a glove requires associating the "thwack" sound of a successful catch with motor actions that control the glove's inertia. The cerebellum handles these complex associations.

• The *amygdala* plays a major role in arousal, orienting the brain to place emphasis on events that are especially important.

• The *thalamus* is a major gateway that filters all sensorimotor input and output to the cortex.

1.2.2 Maps

The most studied part of the brain is the cortex. The two hemispheres of the cortex form a hierarchical memory system. At the lower levels of the memory are simple representations of the sensory input and motor output. Higher levels represent abstract features of the same that are used for problem-solving and control functions. In vision, for example, the lowest part of the cortical hierarchy represents "edges," local sites of abrupt photometric change in the image encoded by the retinas. The highest parts of that same hierarchy represent features of faces, such as emotions and identity. The cortices form a two-dimensional layered sheet of nerve cells that can be grouped together in *maps* wherein cells have common functions. Figure 1.2 shows the basic layout of a monkey cortex that has been flattened to make the map structure more apparent.[10]

1.2.3 Neurons

The major components and cortical maps are architectural features that show up at large and intermediate scales, respectively. A much more stun-

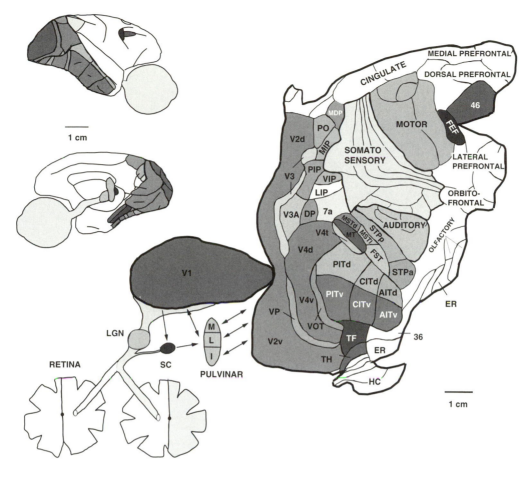

Figure 1.2 The brain's main memory system is the cortex, a two-dimensional multilayered sheet of cells that appears in folds directly underneath the skull. These are specialized into different functions that are laid out in two-dimensional "maps" or collections of cells that can be associated with distinct functions. Although such functional interpretations are constantly being refined and revised, the major areas are as shown. (From Van Essen, Anderson, and Felleman, 1992.)

ning feature shows up at a small scale, and this is the brain's capacity for huge amounts of parallel computation by means of nerve cells, or *neurons*. Neurons come in a small variety of basic shapes, but the main type used for communicating over distances is the pyramidal cell, whose principal features are shown in Figure 1.3.[11] Each of the approximately 10^{11} cortical neurons connects to 10^4 others. This connectivity is nothing short of amazing owing to the special "tree" shape of a neuron. Consider that it is not unusual for a neuron, whose cell body is about 10 microns, or 10^{-5} meters, to connect to neurons one centimeter distant. If the cell body were the size of a marble, its axon would stretch 30 feet. This axon branches more than 10,000 times in the course of making connections,[12] and each one of these branches is capable of sending the cell's signals, which are in the form of voltage spikes. At the end of each axonal branch, the signal is transmitted

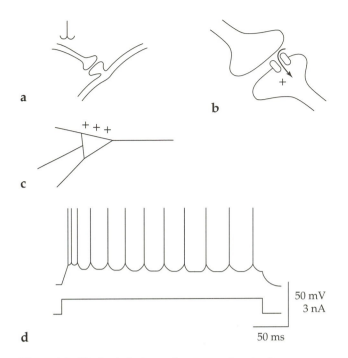

Figure 1.3 The basic features of a neuron showing how a neuron communicates: (*a*) an incoming voltage spike arrives at a synapse; (*b*) this causes ions to flow across the synaptic junction, charging the cell body; (*c*) when sufficient charge has accumulated, the cell fires its own voltage spike. (*d*) Typical spike sequences from a cortical cell. (From Connors and Gutnick, 1990.)

to another cell by *neurotransmitters*, chemical messengers that effect a charge transfer. The site of transfer is called a *synapse*. Synapses on the receiving cell are located on *dendrites*, extensions of the cell near the cell body. In the learning algorithms that are the focus of natural computation, synapses are the central feature, as modulating their efficacy is thought to be the principal way brain programs are constructed.

Think of each neuron as a processor that can compute in parallel with all the other neurons. If the computation could be optimally distributed over these processors, then potential speedups on the order of the number of neurons could be achieved. This speedup is vital because the brain is under even more severe constraints than silicon computers, since its basic computing units—neurons—are more than one million times slower than silicon circuitry.

1.3 COMPUTATIONAL THEORY

If the brain is performing computation, it should obey the laws of computational theory. These results come from two areas, *computability* and *complexity*, and can be paraphrased respectively as follows: (1) You cannot compute nearly all the things you want to compute. (2) The things you can compute are too expensive to compute.

Computability seeks to characterize the entities that can be computed. Computation can be modeled on a universal machine, called a Turing machine. Such a machine has a very simple specification, as shown in Figure 1.4. The machine works by being in a "state" and reading a symbol from linear tape. For each combination of state and tape symbol, the machine has an associated instruction that specifies a triple consisting of the new state, a symbol to write on the tape, and a direction to move. Possible motions are one tape symbol to the left or right. Although the Turing machine operation appears simple, it is sufficiently powerful that if a problem can be solved by any computer it can be solved by a Turing machine.

The things that Turing machines compute are called *computable functions*, and from examining the power of Turing machines, you can learn

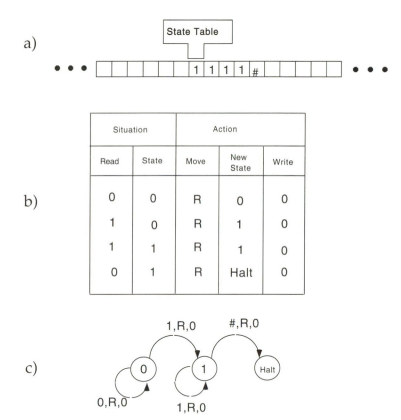

Figure 1.4 (*a*) A Turing machine consists of a linear tape containing a discrete set of symbols. The machine reads the symbol immediately below the tape reader head and, depending on its state, writes a symbol and moves one tape space to the left or right. A Turing machine is completely characterized by its state transition diagram. This example shows a very simple program for erasing a block of contiguous ones. (*b*) The program can be represented by a table that shows what to do for each state and input. (*c*) Equivalently, a Turing machine program can be described by a state transition diagram in which the nodes of a graph are states and arcs are labeled by the symbol read, the direction of motion, and the symbol written. Despite the extreme modesty of its structure, a Turing machine is sufficiently powerful to be able to emulate all the operations of any other computer, albeit much less efficiently.

properties of these functions. The most essential property stems from the fact that Turing machines can be enumerated in correspondence with the integers. Thus the only computable functions are those that can also be put in correspondence with the integers, a countable infinity. This is indeed a limitation since the set of *all* functions can be put in correspondence with the real numbers, an uncountable infinity. Thus there is an uncountably infinite number of uncomputable functions. This is not hard to show formally. Putting the Turing machines in correspondence with the integers only requires that you do not use up the integers too fast, and is left as an exercise. Showing that the integers and reals cannot be put into correspondence can be done by assuming the contrary and then showing that such an assumption leads to a contradiction. First you hypothesize that it can be done for the real numbers between zero and one, and then you find other real numbers that have been left off the list, as shown in Figure 1.5. Therefore, it cannot be done. Hence Turing machines must operate within this limitation.

Complexity seeks to characterize the *cost* of computer algorithms. The way this cost is measured is as a function of the size of the input. For example, sorting a list of n numbers takes time proportional to $n \log n$. Multiplying two square matrices together, each of size $n \times n$, takes time proportional to $n^{\log 7}$. These two examples are regarded as "easy" because their run time is bounded by a polynomial function of their input; that is, you can find a constant k such that the run time $T(n) \le k f(n)$ where $f(n)$ is a polynomial function of n.

Unfortunately for most of the interesting computable problems that have a "best" answer, complexity theory tells us that the cost of computing

Integers	Real Numbers between 0 and 1
1	.0XXXXXXXXXX...
2	.X3XXXXXXXXX...
3	.XX8XXXXXXXX...
4	.XXX2XXXXXXX...
5	.XXXX1XXXXXX...
6	.XXXXX3XXXXX...
.	.
.	.
.	.

Figure 1.5 A hypothetical experiment that will not work. Suppose that the integers can be put in one-to-one correspondence with the real numbers between zero and one. In this example Xs are used to stand for arbitrary digits. Now one can make a new real number that is not on the list by making it differ from the first number in the first significant digit, the second number in the second significant digit, and so on. Therefore, it cannot be on the list.

Table 1.2 Time to solve a problem on a computer that takes 10^{-7} seconds per unit input as a function of the size of the input and the complexity of the algorithm. Times are in seconds except where noted. For *polynomial* complexity functions such as n and n^3, the times remain reasonable. *Exponential* complexity functions such as 2^n and 3^n can only be solved for very modest n.

Algorithmic Complexity	Input Size, n			
	10	30	50	70
n	10^{-6}	3×10^{-6}	5×10^{-6}	7×10^{-6}
n^3	10^{-4}	0.27×10^{-2}	0.12×10^{-1}	0.34×10^{-1}
2^n	0.2×10^{-4}	61 hr	29×10^{13} yr	14×10^{32} yr
3^n	0.18×10^{-1}	15×10^9 yr	47×10^{29} yr	49×10^{60} yr

this answer is prohibitively expensive, since the run time scales as an exponential function of the size of the input, that is,

$$T(n) = kC^n$$

It does not matter what the constants C and k are, so suppose $k = 1$ and $C = 10$. Then if a problem of size 100 can be solved in one second, a problem of size 10,000 would take 10^{100} seconds, or much longer than the age of the universe. Table 1.2 shows additional calculations, revealing the sharp boundary that separates problems that have polynomial run-time functions and problems that have exponential run-time functions. Most interesting problems have exponential worst-case functions, so that the solutions to their worst-case exemplars, for all but the smallest problem sizes, are too expensive to compute.

1.4 ELEMENTS OF NATURAL COMPUTATION

The result of computability theory is fundamental. But the result of complexity theory turns on a series of assumptions that range from the architecture of the machine to the size of the problems to be solved to the criterion to be used in evaluating solutions. Natural computation breaks with all these assumptions and replaces them with a new modeling perspective. The elements of this perspective are as follows:

• *Minimum description length.* The only answers that are practical to compute are those that retreat from the best answer in some sense. Answers can be just good, approximately correct, or correct to a certain probability. A universal metric for all these approximations is the minimum-description-length principle, which measures the cost of encoding regularity in data.

• *Learning.* Biological systems can amortize the cost of algorithms over their lifetime by learning from examples. Such learning can be seen as the "online" detection of regularity. The crucial component of this online performance is the ability to *predict* future events, an ability that has enormous survival value.

• *Specialized architectures.* The massively parallel organization of the brain's neurons can compensate dramatically for their millisecond speeds. Particularly if the input is bounded at some fixed size, as it is with a retina or cochlea, then it can be very cost effective to design special-purpose architectures. In addition, to manage complexity the brain has evolved many hierarchical structures.

These broad elements have led to the development of a wide range of computational models that both are effective and provide many new insights into the possible mechanisms of brain computation. These models lie properly at the boundary of mathematics, computer science, psychology, and neuroscience. Let us elaborate.

1.4.1 Minimum Description Length

Although the results from complexity theory on computational cost are daunting, the key caveat is that they are for the "worst-case" assumptions. Worst-case assumptions mean that the very best result is to be guaranteed, regardless of the difficulty of any particular data set. Figure 1.6 shows that instances of a problem can vary hugely in difficulty. In the traveling salesman problem the challenge is to find the shortest tour of n cities, returning to the point of origin. As the figure shows, some problems are easy enough that very good solutions can be found readily, whereas others may be so difficult that they require testing all possible routes.

Retreating from this standard in any of several directions makes computation practical. For example, the solution may be close to the optimum in cost, but not the best. In the traveling salesman problem, a tour with a length within 10% of the shortest length may do. Another way of reducing cost is to have a solution that has a high probability of being the best, but may not actually be the best. Yet another way of approximating is to have

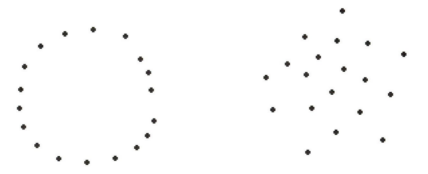

Figure 1.6 Easy (*left*) and difficult (*right*) traveling salesman problems. Finding the minimum tour of the cities can require examining all possible tours in the general case, but getting within a percentage of the best tour is inexpensive in both cases.

a solution that is almost correct. In a biological system that takes time to implement solutions, a partial solution may be satisfactory, as the rest can be filled in later on.

Approximate solutions are almost forced on biological systems because they have to act continuously in the world, and new solutions have to be found by experimentation, either directly or by mental simulation. Since the experimental trials cannot be guaranteed to be the best, the system will necessarily be suboptimal. In the words of Stephen Jay Gould: "In order to be adaptable, an organism must be suboptimal."[13]

In thinking about approximate algorithms it is important to consider their physical embodiment. Something as ordinary as a table might be thought of as running an algorithm that adjusts its atoms continually, governed by an energy function. Whatever its variables are, just denote them collectively by x. Then you can think of the table as solving the problem of adjusting its atoms so as to minimize energy, that is,

$$\min_x E(x)$$

Is this computation? It turns out that it is tricky to say. Some contend that computation is not a *natural kind*,[14] that is, whether or not some device is doing computation depends on the goals of an external observer. This may turn out not to be the case. Extraordinary progress is being made by casting computation in terms of an optimization problem in which some function of the variables of the system is to be minimized. Exploring possible functions is in large part what this book is about.

One of the most promising cost functions views the brain's algorithms as compact codes. This idea stems from the work of Kolmogorov[15] in the 1930s. Consider that a system can always be defined in terms of the sets of input/output data it produces. If these sets are random, then it turns out that this is the best one can do. That is, there is no smaller description of the data than the data itself. However, physical systems incorporate many regularities, and, as a consequence, much more economical descriptions are possible. In particular, small descriptions are created by the brain's encoding mechanisms.

When counting the size of encoded data to see that you really made a net improvement, you have to count the size of the encoder as well. For animals, the encoders are in the form of their behavioral programs. Thus a new version of Occam's razor is that the complexity of a theory (read: corpus of behavioral programs) can be measured in terms of the minimum-description-length principle, which counts succinctness in terms of the compactness of the theory in both the data it accounts for and the complexity of the theory itself. The only step left is to specify a currency for this accounting. The standard units for encoding are *bits* from information theory. Informally, you can think of a bit as the amount of information you obtain from learning the result of an experiment with two equally probable outcomes. In these units the MDL principle is easy to express (see box).

> The complexity of a theory is measured in terms of the number of bits to encode the theory + the number of bits to encode the data with the help of the theory.[16]

Let us illustrate this principle with two examples.

Example 1: A Program That Prints 10,000 Ones Suppose the data set is the string of 10,000 ones,[17] that is,

$1111\cdots1$

These can be compressed by using the equivalent program

```
for i=1 to 10,000 do
    print(1)
```

In this example, the "theory" is a simple program that can be described in just a few hundred bits. Once this program has been created, the "data" are compressed into the null set. In more complicated cases, simpler theories can usually be obtained by not trying to predict all the data exactly but leaving an uncompressed part as a residual, as in the next example.

Example 2: A Neuron's Receptive Field The main form of programming is in terms of the modification of a synapse.[18] To see how this works, consider the example of encoding a small patch of an image by a set of model neurons. Although real synapses are complicated, much insight can be had with a simple model in which their effects are just a multiplication of the synaptic strength with the input. That is, if x is the value of the incoming neuron's input, and the weight w models a synapse on the target cell, the effect of the input is wx. In this simple model, the values of a model neuron's synapses play a major role in specifying how it will respond to its input. Its collection of synapses constitutes a code that makes it especially sensitive for inputs that have the same pattern of activity as the strength of the weights. Figure 1.7 shows how this can be done. The responses of a set of neurons constitute a code that takes into account regularities in the visual world to compress the image samples into a much smaller format.

The minimum-description-length principle is a breakthrough because now one can think of a program as a form of code and the job of the brain's self-organization (algorithms) as producing compact codes. You can view behavioral programs as operating with *compressed descriptions* of data. Theories can be rated according to how much they compress the data.

The value of compact codes is evident in the rapid expansion of brain size in hominid evolution, which presumably pays off in increased fitness. To survive, the brain needs to simultaneously respond quickly to situations and have a large repertoire of responses. Both these avenues have to deal with biological constraints. The speed of responses is limited by the

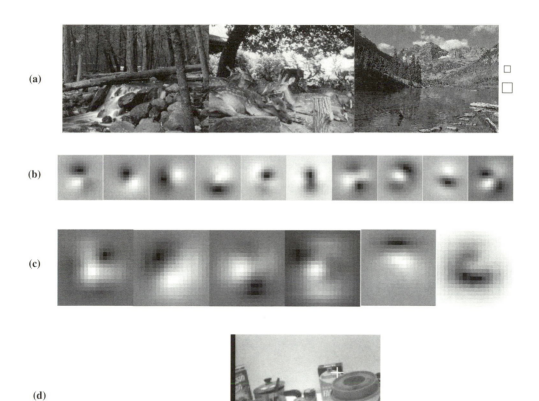

Figure 1.7 How a neuron can represent a code for images. (*a*) 16 × 16 and 20 × 20 sample patches from natural images whose relative size is shown as small boxes on the right are input to 16 neurons' synapses or *receptive fields*. (*b* and *c*) The synapses of 16 model neurons shown with the two receptive field sizes. The weights for the 16 × 16 and 20 × 20 synapses can be both positive and negative numbers. Positive numbers are encoded as lighter squares, and negative numbers are encoded as darker squares. Each of the 16 "neurons" will respond according to how well a particular input matches its receptive field. A collection of such responses constitutes a code that describes the image patch more succinctly than the original samples. (*d*) The portion of a new image centered on the cross to be succinctly encoded as the collective response of 45 such neurons. (*e*) The bars show the firing rate of individual neurons from a horizontal baseline rate. (Parts *d* and *e* are reprinted from *Artificial Intelligence*, 78[12], Rajesh P. N. Rao and Dana Ballard, "An Active Vision Architecture Based on Iconic Representation, p. 473, © 1995 with kind permission of Elsevier Science–NL, Sara Burgerhartstraat 25, 1055 KV Amsterdam, The Netherlands.)

speed of neurons, which cannot signal faster than one millisecond. The size of the repertoire is limited by the number of neurons. (In humans, brain size has exceeded what is practical to push through the birth canal, and flexible skull plates permit postnatal growth of the brain size of up to a factor of four.[19]) Thus the simplest way to improve things is to discover better encodings (algorithms), and the way to measure these is in terms of their information in bits.

It can be extremely disconcerting to think of human attributes such as goals and emotions as being measured and driven by encodings which are in turn measured in bits, but this stance is very helpful if we are to understand the brain. It turns out that goals and emotions can be seen as having essential algorithmic roles in the execution of behaviors.

1.4.2 Learning

Thinking of a program as a form of code and the job of the brain's self-organization (algorithms) as producing compact codes gives you a universal perspective on the brain's algorithms. These are characterized as *learning* algorithms. Kolmogorov complexity provides algorithms with a common task: data compression. The key additional constraint captured by "learning" is that biological algorithms must work *online*. That is, they function continually in the embodiment of the organism. In computer science parlance, they are "anytime" algorithms in that the behaviors must be produced whenever they are needed.

Now consider the principal mechanism of learning. Each of approximately 10^{10} neurons connects to an average of 10^4 other neurons by means of synapses.[20] The principal way of programming the brain is to change the strength of these synapses, as each of the brain's 10^{14} synapses is modifiable. This modifiability gives the brain the capability of continually reprogramming itself to meet current requirements. Learning algorithms exploit this underlying plasticity to amortize the cost of their development. In some cases, this amortization extends far beyond the lifetime of a single individual. This book focuses on three kinds of learning—developmental learning, behavioral learning, and evolutionary learning—all of which affect the architecture of the brain. What distinguishes them is that they operate on very different timescales.

Developmental learning occurs just before and soon after birth and requires on the order of weeks to months. In visual development, for example, stereo vision appears at about five weeks after birth. Most developmental learning occurs in the first year, but complex changes occur on a schedule that continues up to puberty. In terms of brain circuitry, this is the time during which the basic connections are made. The amount of plasticity is enormous. It is estimated that, in the course of searching for the right neural connections, ten times the number of cells that survive puberty are tried out and discarded. The goal of this learning is to process basic stimuli from the environment in order to react quickly. The way this can be done is to associate complex invariants from the environment with actions in a look-up table format. For example, "tiger" has a myriad of sensory instantiations, but the goal is to recognize the essential invariants and associate them with "run!" in the look-up table.

Behavioral learning occurs at the task level. The agent learns to string together primitive physical actions that are encoded in look-up table format to accomplish goals. The key feature of this kind of learning is that the rewards are delayed. Thus the agent has to solve the credit assignment problem: learning which of many different causes at a particular time lead to sources of reward at a later time. Developmental and behavioral learning overlap in time, but developmental learning must occur first, as a set of primitive functions must be in place to get behavioral learning started. Behavioral learning continues throughout one's lifetime.

Evolutionary learning occurs at much longer timescales. By experimenting with the structure of genes, animals can test modifications in architecture. We know that the first bipedal creatures like us appeared about 3 million years ago but that *Homo sapiens* may have appeared as recently as about 200,000 years ago.

Somewhat surprisingly, the resources available to do computation in each of the learning categories are similar. The brain is programmed from experience. At different timescales, experimenters have observed the time needed to acquire certain facilities, so we can estimate an upper bound for the training time for a given level. In general, the bound on the training time T_{train} is given by the simple formula

$$T_{train} = T_p \times N_p$$

where T_p is the time to process stimuli from the environment and N_p is the number of such events required to learn. This formula can be used with the observations of T_{train} from the previous paragraph to estimate the number of presentations for each of the learning types. The results are shown in Table 1.3. What is interesting is that the estimates for N_p are all within a couple of orders of magnitude of each other, indicating that the power of the algorithms is about the same.

Table 1.3 Learning times for human brain processes. Although the timescales of operation are very different, the power of the underlying learning algorithms may be comparable. The power of evolutionary learning is underestimated here, as the search is conducted with a population rather than an individual.

Learning Venue	Exposure Time, T_p	Total Time, T_{train}	Learning Epochs, N_p
Development	10^{-1}	10^7	10^8
Behavior	10^1	10^9	10^8
Evolution	10^{10}	10^{16}	10^6

1.4.3 Architectures

One way of reducing computational cost is to design the computer in such a way as to be specialized for the computations that must be performed. This might seem a violation of the main result of complexity theory: that the cost of an algorithm should be measured only as a function of the size of the input and nothing else. The key difference is that biological systems have finite input sizes. Thus the complexity arguments, which hold in the limit of arbitrarily large inputs, do not necessarily apply. When the input is of finite size, it pays to optimize the machine.[21]

Communicating in physical systems over long distances has costs in time and space.[22] There is great incentive to organize computation so that most of it is done by communicating *locally*, but in any complex system some long-distance communication will be needed. The only way around this problem is to organize such systems hierarchically. This approach allows one to tailor effects so that they can be reliably accessed at the correct temporal and spatial scale. (One can have systems for which local effects can be of great consequence at long scales. Such systems are termed *chaotic*.[23] But these systems cannot be easily utilized in computation.) The bottom line is that for any physical system to be manageable, it must be organized hierarchically.

Constraints of Time and Space Hierarchical systems have a fundamental constraint that stems from the organization of space itself. Whenever a system is constructed of units that are composed of simpler primitives, the more abstract primitives are necessarily larger and slower. The effects of spatial scale are shown in Figure 1.8. Suppose the 0th level of a system is constructed of components of size C that may be thought of as primitives. Then the next level in the system that uses K of these will take up space KC. Moving up the hierarchy, the nth level will cost $K^n C$.

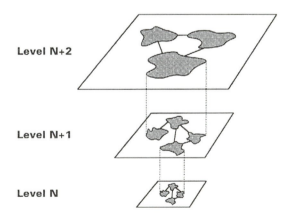

Figure 1.8 Spatial scaling in hierarchical systems. Composite units each take the sum of the space of their components. Thus more abstract circuits necessarily take up more space than their components. (From Newell, 1990.)

Time scales in a similar way, as shown in Figure 1.9, but the reason time may not scale geometrically is that temporal costs can be ameliorated with special algorithms. These usually use special connectivity so as to push temporal costs into the spatial domain. Thus instead of a cost of tM for level n, the actual cost will be T^nM, where $T = f(t)$ is the temporal scaling owing to the special algorithm.

We have just seen that there are fundamental spatiotemporal constraints on hierarchical systems. In a hierarchical system, the more abstract components run slower and take up more space at geometric rates.

Cognitive Hierarchies   The temporal constraints on levels in a hierarchical system can be interpreted in terms of biology.[24] The most fundamental constraint for the human brain is the communication system between neurons. Neurons communicate by sending electrical spikes that take about one millisecond to generate. As a result, the circuitry that uses these spikes for computation has to run slower than this rate. Let us assume that about ten operations are composed at each level. Then local cortical circuitry will require 10 ms. These operations are in turn composed for the fastest "deliberate act." A primitive deliberate act is then 100 ms. Measurements of perception show that such acts take about 50 ms, so the 100-ms estimate is in the ballpark. The next level is the physical act. A primitive physical act might be an eye movement, a hand movement, or a short sentence. Composing these results is a primitive task. A good example is a chess move. Speed chess is played at about 10 seconds per move.[25] Table 1.4 shows these relations.

To summarize the discussion of hierarchies, there are two important points. The first is that the abstract analysis of hierarchical systems finds a reality in the construction of the brain. The evidence is overwhelming that the brain is organized hierarchically. The second point is that the constraints that the individual levels impose on models of computation are quite severe. For example, an eye movement takes about 250 ms (a little shorter than Newell's estimate). To make that movement, the neural machinery must choose the eye-movement target, locate that target in space, and command the eye muscles, all in the time it takes a neuron to send about 100 spikes. This in turn means that many of the operations must be

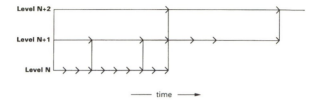

Figure 1.9   Temporal scaling in hierarchical systems. Composite units each take the sum of the time of their components. Thus more abstract operations are necessarily slower than their component operations. (From Newell, 1990.)

Table 1.4 The organization of human computation into temporal bands (after Newell, 1990). Though the cost of developing algorithms may be amortized over a much longer period, ranging from years for developmental learning to centuries for genetic learning, the timescale for their execution is tightly constrained to lie within a range of 100 ms to 10 seconds.

Temporal Scale	Primitive	Example
10 sec	Complex task	Moving in speed chess
2 sec	Simple task	Saying a sentence
300 ms	Physical act	Moving the eyes
50 ms	Neural act	Noticing a stimulus
10 ms	Neural circuit	
1 ms	Neuron spike	

precomputed, as there is not enough time to synthesize elaborate sequences of neural "instructions."

1.5 OVERVIEW

The overall perspective of this book is that learning algorithms develop behavioral programs. Such algorithms can be seen as being driven by the minimum-description-length principle. The brain works to improve its owner's chances of survival by working simultaneously to increase the speed of execution of its programs and the size of its behavioral repertoire.

This book brings together three main types of learning algorithms: neural networks, reinforcement learning, and genetic algorithms. These algorithms operate at very different timescales, but they share a common theme in that they are all optimization algorithms that try to find good solutions to problems using examples as input. Although these algorithms can be useful in many situations, much leverage is gained by studying them as models of brain computation. Thus developmental learning is developed with the objective of encoding quick reactions to stimuli. Reinforcement learning is developed with respect to the brain's problem of using secondary rewards. Genetic algorithms are developed in the context of searching the space of brain architectures. Table 1.5 shows the correspondence used in this text.

Table 1.5 The correspondence between learning algorithms and learning systems in the brain.

Biological Timescale	Computational Model	Function
Development	Neural networks	Memories
Behavior	Reinforcement learning	Programs
Evolution	Genetic algorithms	Architectures

The structure of the book has four parts: a set of core concepts (Part I), followed by the study of the learning algorithms in three settings of increasing abstraction: memories (Part II), programs (Part III), and architectures (Part IV).

1.5.1 Core Concepts

The central ideas of natural computation can be understood in terms of the composition of five basic mathematical and computational ideas: (1) fitness, (2) programs, (3) data, (4) dynamics, and (5) optimization.

• *Fitness.* The brain has to run without a *deus ex machina*, but nonetheless there must be a principle that produces the observed structures and behaviors. Such a principle is that of minimum description length, which captures the survival values of having good models.

• *Programs.* A fundamental concept is that of the brain's internal model of a computation. A very useful model contains two elements: *states* that represent abstractions of the current situation, and *operators,* or actions that govern transitions between states.

• *Data.* State spaces cannot be created out of whole cloth, but must be distilled from multidimensional sensory data. Continuous state spaces can be analyzed for useful structure in sensory data.

• *Dynamics.* A physical system's state has an associated *dynamics.* That is, the state vector changes in time. Such a trajectory is best described differentially in terms of the rate of change of the state vector with time. The easiest systems to deal with are *linear systems.* Such systems are completely characterized by their *eigenvalues* and *initial conditions.* Nonlinear systems can be approximated by linear systems local to stable equilibrium points, or *attractors.*

• *Optimization.* Given the shape of state spaces and the local evolution of trajectories in those spaces, one still needs a way of ranking the desirability of such spaces or trajectories. Ranking requires the ideas of optimization theory, which specifies ways of scoring state space trajectories as well as ways of using the scoring, or *objective function,* to find good paths.

1.5.2 Learning to React: Memories

Memories, or "look-up tables," are a way of storing precomputed correct reactions to situations. A stimulus pattern is sensed, and a response can be generated immediately. The main way of creating such associations is by learning from examples.

• *Content-addressable memory.* Content-addressable memory (CAM) is the principal kind of memory that the brain might have. Its central feature is that the content of a memory also serves as the address for its access. Such memories can be recovered even when they are distorted or have missing parts. The job of a CAM is to fill in the missing parts appropriately. In simple CAMs all the neurons are stimulus driven.

• *Supervised learning.* Simple CAM memories may have trouble making fine distinctions. Remedies for this limitation are to add additional *internal* neurons and train the resultant network with a supervisory signal. The best of the supervised methods uses an error function between the classification produced by the network and the desired classification to improve the classification incrementally.

• *Unsupervised learning.* Supervised learning is an attractive model only in restricted circumstances. For most biological systems, unsupervised learning models that have internal neurons must also be used. These are predominantly stimulus driven, and the prototypes formed are functions of the data distribution of patterns.

1.5.3   Learning During a Lifetime: Programs

Look-up tables can be seen as defining primitive operations that can be composed to form larger behaviors. At the next level these neural primitives can be composed to direct the physical system in the course of more complex behaviors. Such compositions may be thought of as programs. A key feature of such programs is that initially the value of running the program cannot be assumed to be known at every step. Thus learning programs require dealing with reward that is *delayed*. To handle these delays, programs learn to form a *secondary reward function* that estimates future primary reward.

• *Markov systems.* The problem defined by any agent is not only to define a problem state space but also to define a model that expresses the transitions between different states. An extremely general way of performing this task that handles uncertainty is to allow probabilistic transitions between states. Such a system is called a *hidden Markov model.* The use of the word "hidden" signifies that the real states of the world are not known, and that the model states are therefore estimates.

• *Reinforcement learning.* Hidden Markov models (HMMs) provide the necessary substrate for describing reinforcement learning. Reinforcement learning associates rewards with transitions in HMMs such that paths through the HMM tend to maximize reward.

1.5.4   Learning Across Generations: Architectures

Memories and reinforcement strategies can reconfigure the existing structures but cannot alter the hardware design. For that purpose, genetic changes are needed. Genetic algorithms model the alteration of the genes during reproduction in order to create new architectural forms. These algorithms can be understood as experimenting with brain hardware. The basic combination of reproduction and fitness as measured by the organisms' environment ensures that good features tend to spread rapidly throughout the population.

• *Genetic algorithms.* Genetic algorithms are a very abstract model of the process of sexual reproduction within a species' population in which strings of symbols represent the genetic code.

• *Genetic programming.* Biologically, DNA is only part of the story. Proteins must be manufactured that in turn assemble the body structures. In genetic algorithms this process is modeled with the fitness function, which implicitly scores the entire process, even though it is never explicitly represented. In contrast, genetic programs represent individuals as actual programs. The genetic operations are carried out on the actual program code. Consequently, an individual is a functioning program that can be directly tested in the environment.

1.6   THE GRAND CHALLENGE

At the beginning of the decade of the 1990s, scientists were asked to make a list of the problems that could be solved by spectacular advances in computing. Surprisingly, the challenge of understanding the brain with computational models is on the list only peripherally as "vision" and "speech." This reluctance to see computation as central justifiably reflects the immaturity of this endeavor. At this point computational models have not had the spectacular successes of the models of chemistry and physics. But the promise is there. To go further we must understand the computational framework with sufficient clarity in order to ask the right questions. The goal of this book is to further this process.

NOTES

1. From the introduction (by Eric Kandel) to Eric R. Kandel, James H. Schwartz, and Thomas M. Jessell, eds., *Principles of Neural Science,* 3rd ed. (Norwalk, CT: Appleton and Lange, 1991).

2. Patricia S. Churchland and Terrence J. Sejnowski, *The Computational Brain* (Cambridge, MA: MIT Press, 1992); Francis Crick, *The Astonishing Hypothesis: The Scientific Search for the Soul* (New York: Maxwell Macmillan International, 1994).

3. Roger Penrose, *The Emperor's New Mind: Concerning Computers, Minds, and the Laws of Physics* (Oxford: Oxford University Press, 1989).

4. D. A. Pomerleau, "Efficient Training of Artificial Neural Networks for Autonomous Navigation," *Neural Computation* 3 (1991):88–97.

5. G. Tesauro and T. J. Sejnowski, "A Parallel Network that Learns to Play Backgammon," *Artificial Intelligence Journal* 39 (1989):357–90.

6. Whitman Richards, ed., *Natural Computation* (Cambridge, MA: MIT Press, 1988).

7. Ibid., introduction.

8. Churchland and Sejnowski, *The Computational Brain.*

9. The figure is from *Review of Neuroscience* by Ben Pansky and Delmas J. Allen (New York: Macmillan, 1980). The designations of function in the caption are tentative, as the overall operation of the brain circuitry at this scale is far from determined; however, the descriptions are fairly commonly accepted (Kandel, Schwartz, and Jessell, *Principles of Neural Science*).

10. The figure is from David C. Van Essen, Charles H. Anderson, and Daniel J. Felleman, "Information Processing in the Primate Visual System: An Integrated Perspective," *Science* 255 (24 January 1992): 419–23.

11. The part of the figure showing the neural spike train is from B. W. Connors and M. J. Gutnick, "Intrinsic Firing Patterns of Diverse Neocortical Neurons," *Trends in Neurosciences* 13 (1990):98–99.

12. Compare axons to silicon gates, which normally connect to fewer than 10 other gates. Such connectivity would be impossible in silicon without dedicated hardware to specially manage the connections owing to the capacitance of the wires, but biological axons are specially designed to actively propagate the signal without loss.

13. Stephen Jay Gould, "The Basis of Creativity in Evolution" (presentation, Rochester Conference on Creation, University of Rochester, January 1987).

14. Churchland and Sejnowski, *The Computational Brain*.

15. A. N. Kolmogorov and V. A. Uspenskii, "Algorithms and Randomness," *Theory of Probabilities and its Applications* 32–33 (1987):425–55.

16. Jorma Rissanen, *Stochastic Complexity in Statistical Inquiry* (River Edge, NJ: World Scientific, 1989).

17. This example is from Ming Li and Paul Vitányi's standard text, *An Introduction to Kolmogorov Complexity and Its Applications* (New York: Springer-Verlag, 1993).

18. First suggested by Donald O. Hebb in *The Organization of Behavior: A Neuropsychological Theory* (New York: Science Editions, 1949).

19. In contrast, the chimpanzee brain is 80% of its final size at birth. Christopher Wills, *The Runaway Brain: The Evolution of Human Uniqueness* (New York: Basic Books, 1993).

20. Steven Rose, *The Making of Memory: From Molecules to Mind* (New York: Doubleday, Anchor Books, 1992).

21. This point is dramatically made in silicon circuitry in the form of special digital signal-processing chips that can process a video frame in just a fraction of the frame time. This ability has allowed the development of real-time computer vision algorithms for the first time.

22. The ideas in this section were originally developed by Allen Newell in his book *Unified Theories of Cognition* (Cambridge, MA: Harvard University Press, 1990).

23. Gregory L. Baker and Jerry P. Gollub, *Chaotic Dynamics: An Introduction* (New York: Cambridge University Press, 1990).

24. Newell, *Unified Theories of Cognition*.

25. Another reason that the modeling methods here are different from traditional symbol manipulation in AI is that the timescales are much shorter, too short to form a symbol.

EXERCISES

1. Comment on the use of simple models to describe complex structures, giving examples from different fields of cases where such models have proven useful and others where they have not.

2. Estimate the total length of axonal "wiring" in the brain in kilometers (a) assuming that the length of an axon is 0.1 mm, and (b) assuming the length of an axonal *branch* is .01 mm.

3. Derive a scheme to put Turing machines in correspondence with the integers. That is, given a Turing machine's state table, your job is to specify a unique integer that describes it.

4. It is known that humans can react to a visual input and push a button within 400 ms. Given that the visual input from the retina is carried by 1 million neurons, what does this suggest about the average complexity of the algorithm that the brain is using?

5. Given that the effects of incoming voltage signals take 10 ms to make a target cell fire, and that the signals travel at 1 meter/second, estimate the number of sequential synapses that could be involved in the 400-ms reaction of the previous problem.

6. A précis of Roger Penrose's book appears in *Behavioral and Brain Sciences* (Volume 13, 1990, pages 643–705), with commentaries on his position. After digesting the article and one or more of the commentaries, write your own commentary.

I   Core Concepts

The central ideas of natural computation can be understood in terms of the composition of five basic mathematical and computational ideas: (1) fitness, (2) programs, (3) data, (4) dynamics, and (5) optimization.

• *Fitness.* The brain has to run without a *deus ex machina*, but nonetheless there must be a principle that produces the observed structures and behaviors. Such a principle is that of *minimum description length*, which captures the survival values of having good models. A good model consists of behavioral programs that help their owner. To be helpful the corpus of programs should execute quickly and cover as many situations as practical. The minimum-description-length principle measures both execution speed and repertoire. It balances the helpfulness of the programs, in terms of the degree of succinctness of their operations, against their size or internal coding cost.

• *Programs.* A fundamental concept is that of the brain's internal model of a computation. An abstract model contains states and operators that govern transitions between states. Exploring how the states-and-operators model is used to solve well-defined problems, including game playing, is a way of introducing these abstract notions.

• *Data.* The brain's internal states cannot be created out of whole cloth, but must be distilled from sensory data using the minimum-description-length principle. Sensory data form multidimensional state spaces whose essential structure can be described by *eigenvectors* and *eigenvalues*. These address the fundamental problem of determining what aspects of the dimensions are essential and what are not by looking for covariations in data. Eigenvectors and eigenvalues work for linear state spaces, but when the underlying constraints are nonlinear, they are also useful as local approximations.

• *Dynamics.* A physical system's state most often has an associated *dynamics* owing to the fact that it is constructed from physical material that must obey Newton's laws. As a consequence, the range of the state vector describing the brain's program is not random but forms a continuous trajectory in state space. This trajectory is best described differentially in terms of the rate of change of the state vector with time. The easiest systems to deal with are *linear systems*. Such systems are completely characterized by their *eigenvalues* and *initial conditions*. Nonlinear systems can be approximated by linear systems local to stable equilibrium points, or *attractors*.

• *Optimization.* The mathematics of eigenspaces describes the shape of state spaces and the local evolution of trajectories in those spaces, but does not provide any way of ranking the desirability of such spaces or trajectories. Ranking requires the ideas of optimization theory, which specifies ways of scoring state space trajectories as well as ways of using the scoring, or *objective function*, to find good paths. Optimization problems can be solved in two distinct ways. (1) The method of Lagrange multipliers can be used to deal with the constraint imposed by the system dynamics and results in a multidimensional optimization problem that can be solved by classical methods of calculus. (2) The method of dynamic programming allows the optimization equations to be solved directly but at considerable cost.

2 Fitness

ABSTRACT Finding good programs requires a fitness function that evaluates their relative efficacy. A general principle for choosing fitness functions is that of *minimum description length,* or *MDL,* which balances the cost of the programs against their cost in terms of describing data using the program. This cost can be measured using the tools of *information theory.*

2.1 INTRODUCTION

The task of analyzing the brain's programs is succinctly introduced by Nicholls et al.

The brain uses stereotyped electrical signals to process all the information it receives and analyzes. The signals are symbols that do not resemble in any way the external world they represent, and it is therefore an essential task to decode their significance.[1]

Good programs can quickly recognize or classify data into situations that have been previously encountered. When those data show up, the animal knows what to do. Think of the program as a *code* for the data that represents the behavior that is appropriate given particular data. The value of short codes for programs is enormous. Shorter programs expand the behavioral repertoire and allow faster decisions.

That data are compressed in behavioral programs is illustrated by an example of insect behavior.[2] Ants were allowed to search mazes in the form of a binary tree, as shown in Figure 2.1. Each maze had food at just one of the ends. Once an ant had learned the location of the food in a particular maze, it then communicated that location to another ant at the beginning of the maze. The time needed to do so was compared for different food locations from different trials. The results are shown in Table 2.1. If the ants had a literal code for turns, one would expect the time to communicate to be proportional to the number of turns. The interesting result is that paths that have a regular structure require shorter times to communicate, implying that the ants are using a compressed code for them.

An essential part of guiding data compression is the choice of a heuristic function, or *fitness function,* that rates the value of different programs. Many fitness functions are possible, and which fitness functions are used by the brain is an open question. While we may not be able to pin down the

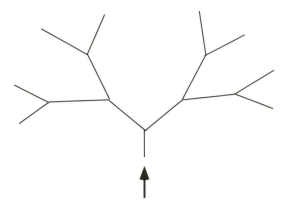

Figure 2.1 The binary tree maze (constructed from matches). (Adapted from Reznikova and Ryabko, 1986.)

Table 2.1 Data showing the communication times for paths in mazes. (From Reznikova and Ryabko, 1986.)

Number	Sequence of Turns to Food	Average Time (Seconds)	Sample Standard Deviation	Number of Tests
1	LLL	72	8	18
2	RRR	75	5	15
3	LLLLLL	84	6	9
4	RRRRR	78	8	10
5	LLLLL	90	9	8
6	RRRRRR	88	9	5
7	LRLRLR	130	11	4
8	RLRLRL	135	9	8
9	LLR	69	4	12
10	LRLL	100	11	10
11	RLLLR	120	9	6
12	RRLRL	150	16	8
13	RLRRRL	180	20	6
14	RRLRRR	220	15	7
15	LRLLRL	200	18	5

ingredients of the brain's fitness functions, we can in broad outline develop the basis from which such functions are likely to be constructed. The essential idea is that one would like to extract the regularities in data. Where such regularities exist, the data can be encoded or compressed. *Information theory* provides a basis for doing so.

Information theory is about codes. Objects in the world are not directly observable but are necessarily encoded in sensory data. Communicating such data efficiently, whether externally by spoken or written symbols, or internally by signals sent from neuron to neuron in the brain, requires compact codes. And as just mentioned, a program may be thought of as a compact way of encoding the data it operates on. Two problems in developing codes are (1) dealing with noise that corrupts the signal and (2) making the codes compact so that they can be transmitted quickly. Information theory describes metrics for measuring codes that address both of these problems.

Information theory is a natural for dealing with programs encoded in terms of neurons for several reasons. First of all, its units—"bits"—are about making decisions, as are programs. Second, almost all of the brain's 10^{11} neurons have the same signaling mechanism, communicating with digital spikes. And third, these spikes are noisy and slow, so that reliability and fast transmission are important issues.

2.2 BAYES' RULE

The cornerstone of information theory is *probability theory*, which characterizes uncertainty. For a brushup on probability theory, see the appendix to this chapter. We will start with probability theory's main inference rule, *Bayes' rule*, which allows the interrelation of different hypotheses. Bayes' rule is a model of the world, but not the only one; there are several other ways of modeling probabilistic inference.[3] However, Bayes' has become standard, spurred by the elegant use of networks to keep track of the relationships between different hypotheses.[4]

The centerpiece of probabilistic reasoning is the calculation of the probability of a conditional event, $P(A \mid B)$, read as "the probability of A given that B happened." This can be expressed in terms of the ratio of other probabilities in Bayes' rule as

$$P(A \mid B) = \frac{P(A, B)}{P(B)}$$

Figure 2.2 motivates this rule using Venn diagrams. Given that B occurred, the right thing to do is to renormalize the universe so that the probability of A occurring is expressed as a fraction of B's area.

An extremely important setting for Bayes' rule is that of *maximum likelihood*. In this setting the goal is to calculate the probability of a hypothesis or model M, given data D, or

$$\max_{M} P(M \mid D)$$

This rule is very natural and intuitive, but the probability $P(M \mid D)$ is typically difficult to measure. It is much easier to obtain *a priori* distributions $P(D \mid M)$. These can be related to *a posteriori* distributions $P(M \mid D)$ by Bayes' rule: $P(M \mid D) = \frac{P(D \mid M)P(M)}{P(D)}$. It is assumed that all the terms on the right-hand side (RHS) can be measured ahead of time or from on-line exemplars. The term $P(D \mid M)P(M)$ is the probability or *likelihood* that the data was produced by model M. Assigning it so is using the maximum likelihood rule.

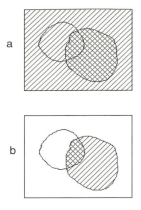

Figure 2.2 (*a*) Using the Venn diagram, the probability of an event *B* can be thought of as the ratio of the area allocated to *B* scaled by the area allocated to the universal event *U*. (*b*) Bayes' rule works similarly. Once it is known that *B* occurred, the appropriate area for the event *A* is given by *A* ∩ *B* and the appropriate area of the new universe is now that of *B*.

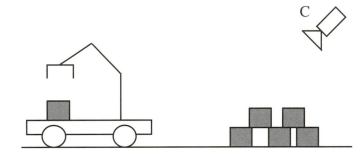

Figure 2.3 A setting for the use of Bayes' rule. A robot picks up boxes aided by data from a camera (C).

Example: Vision Test A robot's job is to pick up boxes and take them to a designated location (Figure 2.3). However, the robot's picking-up device is faulty and works only with probability 0.8. If the robot turns up without a box, it is sent back for another try. You decide to install a camera to test whether a box has been picked up. Let '*B*' represent the datum that the camera test reports the box picked up and *B* be the hypothesis that it is actually picked up. The specifications for the camera are in terms of its conditional *a posteriori* probability distribution:

	'*B*'	¬'*B*'
B (box picked up)	$P('B' \mid B) = 0.9$	$P(\neg'B' \mid B) = 0.1$
¬*B* (box not picked up)	$P('B' \mid \neg B) = 0.2$	$P(\neg'B' \mid \neg B) = 0.8$

Presumably these data are obtained through many tests.

If the camera test says the box was picked up, what is the probability that the box was actually picked up? To solve this problem you would like to know $P(B \mid {'B'})$. This can be obtained from the Bayes inversion formula:

$$P(B \mid {'B'}) = \frac{P({'B'} \mid B)P(B)}{P({'B'})}$$

where $P({'B'})$ can be computed from

$$P({'B'}) = P({'B'}, B) + P({'B'}, \neg B)$$

So that

$$P(B \mid {'B'}) = \frac{P({'B'} \mid B)P(B)}{P({'B'}, B) + P({'B'}, \neg B)}$$

$$= \frac{P({'B'} \mid B)P(B)}{P({'B'} \mid B)P(B) + P({'B'} \mid \neg B)P(\neg B)}$$

$$= \frac{1}{1 + \frac{P({'B'} \mid \neg B)P(\neg B)}{P({'B'} \mid B)P(B)}}$$

Combining and substituting,

$$P(B \mid {'B'}) = \frac{1}{1 + \frac{(0.2)(0.2)}{(0.9)(0.8)}} = \frac{1}{1.056} \cong 0.95$$

In other words, the camera test has improved the situation: With the test, the robot is sent back only 5% of the time, versus 20% without it.

2.3 PROBABILITY DISTRIBUTIONS

In the foregoing example, the event space is discrete and small scale. But dealing with large systems of neurons requires analyzing large numbers of discrete events and also continuous events. To accomplish this purpose requires the notion of a *probability distribution.*

2.3.1 Discrete Distributions

Discrete events can be described with a probability mass function $P(x)$ that keeps track of the probability associated with each event. It is also useful to know certain features of this function, such as its average value, or *mean,* and the spread, or *variance,* about that value. The standard deviation σ, which is just the square root of the variance, is also useful. The mean may be estimated from n samples of x_i that occur with $P(x)$ as

$$m = \frac{1}{n} \sum_{i=1}^{n} x_i$$

and the variance as

$$\sigma^2 = \frac{1}{n} \sum_{i=1}^{n} (x_i - m)^2$$

Two extremely important probability mass functions have an analytic form. These are the binomial distribution and its approximation for special cases, the Poisson distribution.

Binomial Distribution The starting point for the analysis is a set of n independent experiments, the best example of which is tossing a coin. Suppose that you toss a coin three times. The possible outcomes are

$HHH, HHT, HTH, THH, HTT, THT, TTH, TTT$

Suppose the problem is to find the probability of exactly 0, 1, 2, or 3 heads. In this example it can be done by counting. Thus

$$P(0) = \frac{1}{8}, P(1) = \frac{3}{8}, P(2) = \frac{3}{8}, P(3) = \frac{1}{8}$$

For $P(1)$ the probability of each individual outcome is $\frac{1}{2} \times \frac{1}{2} \times \frac{1}{2} = \frac{1}{8}$, and there are three ways it can happen. In general, if the probability of success is p and that of failure $q = 1 - p$, then the general formula is the binomial distribution given by

$$P(k) = \binom{n}{k} p^k q^{n-k} \qquad (2.1)$$

where $\binom{n}{k}$ is the term that keeps track of all the different ways of getting k "heads" in n tosses of the coin, and is given by

$$\binom{n}{k} = \frac{n!}{k!(n-k)!}$$

The binomial distribution has a mean given by

$m = np$

and a variance given by

$\sigma^2 = npq$

Poisson Distribution The binomial distribution is extremely useful but difficult to calculate, so there is a premium on approximations to it that are easier to compute. The most useful of these is the Poisson distribution, which works when p is small. In this case,

$$\binom{n}{k} p^k q^{n-k} \approx \frac{(np)^k}{k!} e^{-np}$$

The Poisson distribution has a mean given by

$m = np$

and a variance given by

$\sigma^2 = np$

The Poisson distribution is usually used when dealing with events that occur with respect to a continuous quantity, such as length or time. Thus the probability is usually measured as the number of occurrences in a given interval, which in turn is calculated by a rate of occurrence × a reference interval. Letting I be the events per reference interval and N the size of the interval of interest, the formula becomes

$$P(k) = \frac{(NI)^k}{k!} e^{-NI}$$

As an example, if a neuron produces an average of one spike per 100 ms, what is the probability of seeing three spikes in $\frac{1}{4}$ second? Here $I = \frac{1}{100}$ and $N = 250$, so that

$$P(3) = \frac{(2.5)^3}{3!} e^{-2.5} \approx 0.15$$

For the Poisson approximation to work, the rate of occurrence must obey certain properties:

1. For an interval of given length, the frequency with which an event will occur is proportional to the length of the interval.

2. The occurrence of more than one of the events in the interval is rare.

3. The occurrence of an event in one interval is independent of the occurrence of an event in another interval.

2.3.2 Continuous Distributions

In a continuous distribution, a random variable X takes on real values x. In this case it does not make sense to talk about the probability of any specific value, but instead the probability of an interval. The *probability density function* $p(x)$ is defined as the limit of such intervals. Formally,

$$p(x) = \lim_{\Delta x \to 0} \frac{P(x < X \leq x + \Delta x)}{\Delta x}$$

This function is shown in Figure 2.4.

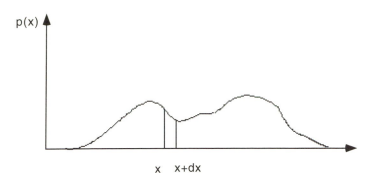

Figure 2.4 The probability of real-valued random variables is defined by intervals denoting area under the density function.

Although a random vector is fully characterized by its density function, such functions are often difficult to determine or mathematically complex to use. This complexity motivates modeling distributions with functions that can be described by a low number of parameters. The most important of such parameters are the continuous versions of the *mean* and *variance*, introduced with discrete distributions.

The mean is defined by

$$m = E\{X\} = \int xp(x)\,dx$$

and the variance by

$$\sigma^2 = E\{(X - M)^2\}$$

Normal Distribution   One of the most useful parametric distributions is the normal distribution or *Gaussian* of a continuous random variable X. It is useful because most observed random variables tend to be the sum of several random components, and the sum of random components tends to be normally distributed.

The normal distribution is given by

$$p(x) = \frac{e^{-\frac{1}{2}d^2(x,\,m,\,\sigma)}}{\sqrt{2\pi\sigma}}$$

where d^2 is given by

$$d^2(x,\,m,\,\sigma) = \frac{(x - m)^2}{\sigma}$$

Especially useful is the cumulative distribution, which is given by

$$\Phi(x) = P(X < x) = \int_{-\infty}^{x} p(u)\,du$$

This distribution can be tabulated for $m = 0$ and $\sigma = 1$, as is done in Table 2.2. When the mean and variance are not zero and one, respectively, the table can still be used, but instead of x you use the argument $(x - m)/\sigma$.

Table 2.2   The integral under the Gaussian probability density function.

x	$\Phi(x)$	x	$\Phi(x)$
0.0	0.500	1.4	0.919
0.2	0.579	1.6	0.945
0.4	0.655	1.8	0.964
0.6	0.726	2.0	0.977
0.8	0.788	2.2	0.986
1.0	0.841	2.4	0.992
1.2	0.885	2.6	0.995

Gaussian Approximation to a Binomial Distribution To see how the cumulative distribution is useful, consider the problem of calculating the probabilities of the binomial distribution when n is large. Using Equation 2.1 involves a lot of calculation. It turns out, however, that the number of successes in a binomial distribution can be approximated with a normal distribution for large n. Let us phrase the question as, Given a set of n trials, what is the probability that the frequency of successes falls between the interval specified by f_1 and f_2? The normal distribution allows the following approximation:

$$\Phi(x_2) - \Phi(x_1) = P(f_1 < X \le f_2) = \frac{1}{\sqrt{2\pi}} \int_{x_1}^{x_2} e^{-\frac{u^2}{2}} \, du$$

where

$$x_1 = \sqrt{\frac{n}{pq}}(f_1 - p)$$

and

$$x_2 = \sqrt{\frac{n}{pq}}(f_2 - p)$$

Example Use the Gaussian approximation to the binomial distribution to estimate $P(k > 27)$ for $n = 50, p = \frac{2}{3}$.

To solve this first use the fact that

$$P(k > 27) = 1 - P(k \le 27)$$

Next, since $f_2 = \frac{k}{n}$, x_2 is given by

$$x_2 = \sqrt{\frac{n}{pq}}(f_2 - p) = \sqrt{\frac{50}{\frac{4}{9}}}\left(\frac{27}{50} - \frac{2}{3}\right) \approx -2$$

So that

$$\Phi(x_2) = \frac{1}{\sqrt{2\pi}} \int_{-\infty}^{x_2} e^{-\frac{u^2}{2}} \, du = 1 - \Phi(-x_2)$$

Interpolating from Table 2.2, $\Phi(2) = 0.98$, so that, putting all this together, the probability of k exceeding 27 is 0.98.

Does this jibe with your intuition? From Table 2.2, $\Phi(0) = 0.5$. This is the result when $f = p$ as you might expect. With an increasing number of samples, it becomes more and more likely that the measured frequency will be close to the mean.

2.4 INFORMATION THEORY

The setting for information theory we will consider is that of communicating a discrete set of symbols.[5] The two principal questions of interest are efficiency and redundancy.

Efficiency is important in the encoding of the symbols. If the codes are inefficient, then the symbol is unnecessarily long and the communication of the message takes more time or more space. An example of this setting is the retina and optic nerve in the human eye. Although there are 10^8 cells in the retina, there are only 10^6 cells in the optic nerve that connects the retina to the rest of the brain. Hence the thought is that the retina encodes the image by removing redundant information prior to the transmission of the code by the optic nerve.[6]

Redundancy is necessary for reliable transmission in the face of noise. An example of this is natural language. On the surface, without considering pronunciation and grammar, there are 26^5 words that are 5 letters long (over 10 million) in the English language, yet the average English vocabulary, even without the five-letter restriction, is only about 5,000 words. Thus the code for English is very redundant, presumably to facilitate language recognition between different speakers.

2.4.1 Information Content and Channel Capacity

Information theory needs a place to put the symbols. This is the *channel*. A channel might be spatial, as in the page of a book, or temporal, as in a slice of time used to broadcast messages.[7]

Let n be the number of discrete symbols $S_1, S_2, ..., S_n$ that can be used, and let m be the length of the message. Then the number of messages is

$$M = n^m$$

The *information capacity* of a channel with n symbols and m locations for symbols is defined as the logarithm of the number of messages. The reason for this definition is the intuition that information should be additive. Doubling the size of the channel should double the amount of information. This leads to

$$C_m = km \ln n$$

where k is a constant of proportionality. The next step is to choose a value for k. To do this the unit of channel capacity is defined as the capacity of a channel, which has just two symbols, thus

$$C_0 = 1 = k \ln 2$$

so that

$$k = \frac{1}{\ln 2}$$

Thus in general,

$$C = \frac{\ln n}{\ln 2} = \log_2 n$$

The dimensionless quantity is nonetheless referred to in terms of "bits."

Table 2.3 Binary encoding for a database of nine names.

Name	Code
Alfie	0000
Brad	0001
Carol	0010
Derek	0011
Edwin	0100
Frank	0101
Greg	0110
Helga	1000
Irene	1001

Now let us turn our attention to the messages that are to be placed in the channel. The information content of a set of N_m messages is defined to be

$$I_m = \log N_m$$

Think of this as the minimum information capacity into which the information can be reversibly encoded assuming all the messages are equally frequent. Naturally in designing a channel you would want the capacity to be greater than the information content of the messages, that is,

$$I_m = \log N_m < C_m$$

To illustrate these concepts, consider the database of nine names shown in the left-hand column of Table 2.3. Using a code of 27 symbols (26 letters plus a blank) and names of length 5 letters allows 27^5 messages. Thus the channel capacity is

$$C_5 = \log 27^5 = 15 \log 3 = 23.78 \text{ bits}$$

It is easy to verify that the channel capacity is adequate for the nine messages:

$$I_m = \log N_m = \log 9 < 23.78$$

Since the information is so much less than the channel capacity, one suspects that the signal could be better encoded. Let's try the 4-bit binary code in Table 2.3. Now the channel capacity is just

$$C = 4 \text{ bits}$$

This is still less than the best code, which could use the beginning letter of each name as a 9-element character set. Then the capacity would be

$$C = \log 9 \text{ bits}$$

2.4.2 Entropy

The foregoing discussion assumes that the channel is being used to send one symbol at a time. The more useful case occurs when the channel is used to send many symbols, where each symbol in the message occurs with a given frequency. For this case we need the concept of *entropy*, or information rate.

Entropy can also be thought of as a measure of the uncertainty of the contents of the message before it has been received. If there are n messages that have frequencies p_i, $i = 1,\dots, n$, then entropy H is defined as

$$H = -\sum_{i=1}^{n} p_i \log p_i \tag{2.2}$$

To motivate this definition, consider the case of a binary channel with only ones and zeros. Further constrain all messages to be of length m and to have exactly m_1 ones and m_2 zeros. Naturally $m_1 + m_2 = m$. The number of different possible messages of this distribution of ones and zeros is just

$$N_m = \binom{m}{m_1} = \frac{m!}{m_1! m_2!}$$

Thus the information in the ensemble of these messages is just

$$I_m = \log N_m = \log m! - \log m_1! - \log m_2!$$

If the m_i, $i = 1, 2$ are so large that $\log m_i \gg 1$, then you can approximate the preceding equation as

$$\log N_m = m \log m - m_1 \log m_1 - m_2 \log m_2$$

So the average information $I = I_m/m$, can be obtained by dividing by m:

$$I = \log m - \frac{m_1}{m} \log m_1 - \frac{m_2}{m} \log m_2$$

This can be rearranged as

$$-\frac{m_1}{m} \log \frac{m_1}{m} - \frac{m_2}{m} \log \frac{m_2}{m}$$

Finally, interpreting $\frac{m_i}{m}$ as the probability p_i leads to

$$I = -\sum_{i=1}^{2} p_i \log p_i$$

which can be generalized to Equation 2.2 for the case of n symbols instead of two. Thus the motivation for interpreting this equation as average information rate. It is also important to understand the relationship between "bits" as used in computers and bits as used in information theory. Suppose that a computer bit can take on the values 0 and 1 with equal probability. In this special case the entropy is

$$H = -\frac{1}{2} \log \frac{1}{2} - \frac{1}{2} \log \frac{1}{2} = 1$$

In other words, one bit in the computer, given equal probabilities, produces one bit of information.

It can be shown that

$$0 \le H \le \log n$$

The lower bound is simply understood. Imagine that the message is known; then for that message, its probability is 1 and the rest are 0. Thus all the terms in the expression are 0, either by virtue of p_i being 0 or the one instance when $\log(1)$ is 0. Thus $0 \le H$. For the upper bound, try to pick the probabilities to maximize H subject to the constraint that the sum of the probabilities is 1, that is, $\sum_{i=1}^{n} p_i = 1$. To do this requires the tools of Chapter 5 (see Problem 5.3), but the answer is that all the probabilities have to be equal, which makes them each $\frac{1}{n}$ so that $H_{max} = \log n$.

In summary, the basic result is that making the codes equally probable maximizes entropy, and this in turn is a measure of coding efficiency.

2.4.3 Reversible Codes

To see how the entropy measure is used, consider a simple example. Suppose that a binary code is used where $P(1) = \frac{7}{8}$ and $P(0) = \frac{1}{8}$. Then in a typical message there should be a preponderance of ones, for example,

11011111111110111111011111111111101 . . .

The capacity for strings of a given length, say the first 21 characters, is just

$$C^{21} = \log 2^{21} = 21 \text{ bits}$$

However, you know that the information is just 21 × the average information per character, or

$$I = \sum_{i=1}^{2} p_i \log p_i = \frac{1}{8} \log \frac{1}{8} + \frac{7}{8} \log \frac{7}{8} = 0.538$$

so that

$$I^{21} = 21 \times 0.538 = 11.30 \text{ bits}$$

The fact that the information is less than the capacity opens up the possibility of shortening the message by using a coding strategy. Now an information rate of $-\sum p_i \log p_i$ is the best we can do. Thus we expect that the average rate (or length) is going to be greater than this—that is, that

$$-\sum p_i \log p_i \le \sum p_i l_i$$

where l_i is the length of the ith code word. From this it is seen that equality occurs when

$$l_i = -\log p_i$$

and this is in fact the best strategy for picking the lengths of the code words.

A very elegant way of choosing code words is to use Huffman coding,[8] which is described as Algorithm 2.1.

Algorithm 2.1 Huffman Coding

1. Divide the data into blocks and generate the probabilities of the blocks according to the product of the probabilities of each of the symbols composing the block.

2. Pick the two smallest probabilities, add them, and record the result as the root of a tree (see Figure 2.5).

3. Repeat this process, using the roots of trees as candidate probabilities along with any remaining code word probabilities.

4. When there is just one root, use the tree to generate the code words.

Suppose you choose blocks of three characters to be encoded. Then the possibilities, along with their probabilities of occurrence, are shown in Table 2.4.

To generate the code words, the two smallest probabilities in the table are summed and form the root of a tree, as shown in Figure 2.5. This process is repeated, as described in the algorithm, until a single tree is formed. Figure 2.6 shows the result of applying the algorithm to the data in Table 2.4. Given that tree, the code words are generated by labeling the left branches of the tree with zeros and the right branches with ones. Next, for each block to be encoded, the concatenation of the symbols on a path from the root to the block is used as the code word. For example, 100 is encoded as 11100.

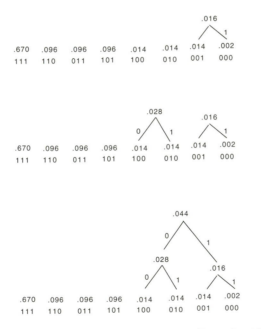

Figure 2.5 Stages in applying the Huffman algorithm. Generating the tree starts by picking the two least probable blocks, which are on the extreme right. Their probabilities sum to .016 and form the root of a subtree. Next the process is repeated, and the subtree with root probability .028 is generated. At this point the two subtree probabilities are smaller than any of the other probabilities, so they form a new subtree. The process terminates when there is only one tree root.

Table 2.4 Huffman encoding for the example.

Block	Probability	Code Word
111	.670	0
110	.096	100
011	.096	101
101	.096	110
100	.014	11100
010	.014	11101
001	.014	11110
000	.002	11111

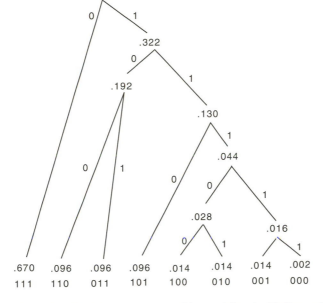

Figure 2.6 The final tree generated by applying the Huffman algorithm. At this point the code words for each block can be generated by traversing the tree. For example, the code word for block 100 is 11100.

Using this code, the first 21 characters of the original string can be encoded as

1000001100100

This result is 13 bits long, which is greater than the expected 11.30, but this difference is just due to the short length of the string.

Irreversible Codes Huffman codes are reversible in that given the code you can recover the original bit sequence. But most biological situations do not require reversible codes and in fact can save many bits by being irreversible. One common situation is that of a prototype, as shown in Figure 2.7. Here it can be the case that just the bits that describe the prototype need be sent, and the individual samples can be described in terms of the

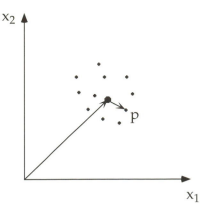

Figure 2.7 An irreversible coding strategy. A single prototype is used to encode all the data points shown. For further information a parametric description of the underlying distribution may be included in the code, but this strategy still results in a huge savings over encoding all the individual points.

underlying probability distribution. When this distribution can be summarized in terms of just a few parameters, as in the case of a Gaussian, it results in a big savings.

2.5 CLASSIFICATION

Now that you have seen how redundancy in a signal can be exploited to produce shorter codes, let us show how lengthening the code can increase reliability. The example we will use is that of encoding prototypes with very long random binary vectors. Consider the case of M prototypes and random vectors of length n where $M \ll 2^n$. It turns out that such vectors have a rather surprising property: as the length n increases, the probability of their being a distance $n/2$ apart goes to one. Here distance between two prototypes is measured as the *Hamming* distance, which is the number of bits that do not match.

Now further suppose that the probability of an error in a bit is p so that the number of errors in the prototypes is binomially distributed. We choose to decide that the input belongs to the prototype if its likelihood ratio is greater than 10^6. From this we can calculate where to put the decision boundary. These steps are shown in Figure 2.8.

Here there are two such prototypes, each with its associated distribution. The *likelihood ratio* for a given measurement x is given by

$$\frac{p(x \mid H_1)}{p(x \mid H_2)}$$

For example, the ratio for $x = 0.8$ is shown marked on the diagram.

As a specific example consider the case where the prototype points have a Gaussian probability density function with variance σ^2. Consider a point that is almost midway between two prototypes but a little toward one of the points by a distance na. Then it is easy to show that the likelihood ratio is given by

$$e^{\frac{n^2 a}{\sigma^2}}$$

This increases dramatically with increasing n, showing the reliability of very long codes in classification. If the measurement is just slightly biased toward a particular prototype, then it becomes overwhelmingly likely that that prototype is the representative.

As shown in Figure 2.9, this approach has been used in a personal identification system based on measurements of the iris pattern of the eye.[9] It turns out that this pattern is unique to every individual, more so than fin-

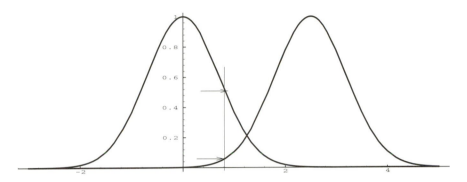

Figure 2.8 The situation when coding prototypes in terms of very long vectors results in having to classify an input vector according to the prototype that is nearest. To make this decision the likelihood ratio (shown by arrows) can be used.

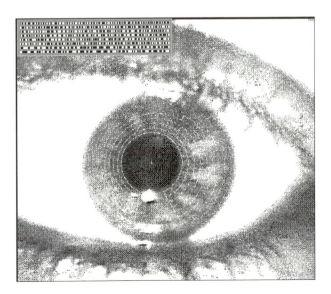

Figure 2.9 An ingenious encoding of the human iris illustrates the virtues of redundant features in decision making. In an annulus around the pupil the pattern of the iris is turned into a bar code that is unique for each individual. (From Daugman; © 1993 IEEE.)

gerprints. Thus 250 measurements of different parts of the iris are sufficient to uniquely classify an individual.

2.6   MINIMUM DESCRIPTION LENGTH

After a lengthy opening development we can now introduce the centerpiece
of this chapter, which is a general way of measuring fitness. Minimum description length (MDL)[10] can be situated in the context of information theory. The idea is that of sending a message that describes a theory. One way
to do so would be just to send all the data, as in a sense this is a literal description of the theory. But the intuition behind Occam's razor is to favor
compact theories. MDL captures this by allowing the message to have the
form of a description of the theory plus a description of the data when encoded by the theory. The assumption is that the sender and receiver agree
on the semantics of a language for the message and the cost is then the
length of the code for the message. Thus the combined length of the message, $L(M, D)$, is a sum of two parts,

$$|L(M, D)| = |L(M)| + |L(D \text{ encoded using } M)|$$

To enflesh this idea further let us approach this problem from the van-
tage point of Bayes' rule. In terms of Bayes' rule, the probability of a model
given data can be expressed as

$$P(M \mid D) = \frac{P(D \mid M)P(M)}{P(D)}$$

Picking the best model can be expressed as maximizing $P(M \mid D)$, or

$$\max_M P(D \mid M)P(M)$$

You do not have to consider $P(D)$ here because it is constant across all
models. Now maximizing this expression is equivalent to maximizing its
logarithm, as the logarithm is monotonic and will not affect the outcome.
So

$$\max_M \left[P(D \mid M)P(M) \right] = \max_M \left[\log P(D \mid M) + \log P(M) \right]$$

and this is the same as minimizing its negative:

$$\min_M \left[-\log P(D \mid M) - \log P(M) \right] \tag{2.3}$$

But now remember the earlier result that for a minimal code that has probability of being sent P, the length of the code is

$$-\log P \tag{2.4}$$

so that using Bayes' rule for the best model selection is equivalent to selecting the MDL model. This is a remarkable result.[11]

When the data are encoded using the model, the parts that are left over
are called the *residuals.* Typically the sum of residuals is a random variable

because if it had a lot of structure, this could be incorporated into the model. Assume the residuals are distributed in the form of a Gaussian with variance a. Then

$$p(D \mid M) = \left(\frac{1}{2\pi a}\right)^{\frac{N}{2}} e^{-\frac{1}{2a}\sum_{i=1}^{n}(x_i - m_i)^2}$$

If in turn the model is a neural network with a set of parameters w_i, $i = 1,\ldots, W$, then we can assume that they also are distributed according to a Gaussian, with variance β. Therefore,

$$p(M) = \left(\frac{1}{2\pi\beta}\right)^{\frac{W}{2}} e^{-\frac{1}{2\beta}\sum_i w_i^2}$$

Substituting these two equations into Equation 2.3,

$$\min_{M} \left[-\log P(D \mid M) - \log P(M)\right] = \frac{1}{2a}\sum_{i=1}^{n}(x_i - m_i)^2 + \frac{1}{2\beta}\sum_i w_i^2 + \text{const.}$$

This equation illustrates the central ideas, namely, that to minimize the code length you should minimize the variance of the residual, and that this term trades off with the cost of the model. This is the reason many neural learning algorithms minimize the sum of the squared error between the prediction of the model, the neural network output, and the desired output. In the case of data points $x_1,\ldots, x_n$ this is

$$\sum_{i=1}^{n}(x_i - m_i)^2$$

where m_i is the network output for data set i. But this is simply proportional to the variance of the residual. Thus minimizing this residual is compatible with using the MDL principle. You will see many other examples of the MDL principle throughout the text, but to get started, consider the following case of having encoded an image with neurons.

Example: Image Coding   Suppose that an image is to be represented with m code neurons that connect to an array of $n \times n$ neurons, as shown in Figure 2.10. Each neuron connects to all the neurons composing the array by way of synapses. Thus the kth code neuron has $n \times n$ synapses w_{ijk}. The MDL principle specifies that the best code will have a combination of a small code length and a small residual. The code length is the number of bits it takes to specify all the r_k's and the number of bits it takes to specify all the w_{ijk}'s. The residual is just the difference between the input image and the reconstruction of the image using the code neurons. The reconstructed image can be specified as

$$I'_{ij} = \sum_{k=1}^{m} w_{ijk} r_k$$

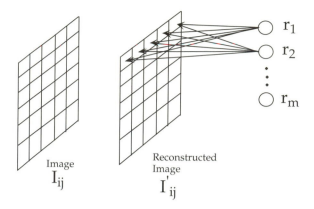

Figure 2.10 The MDL principle applied to image coding. The model is an internal code for an image that is represented by m neurons' responses r_k, $k = 1, ..., m$ together with synapses w_{ijk}, $i = 1, ..., n$; $j = 1, ..., n$; $k = 1, ..., m$. The residual is the squared difference between the original image and the reconstructed image $\sum_{i=1}^{n} \sum_{j=1}^{n} (I_{ij} - I'_{ij})^2$.

and the MDL principle specifies that the r_k's and w_{ijk}'s be chosen to minimize

$$\sum_{i=1}^{n} \sum_{j=1}^{n} (I_{ij} - I'_{ij})^2 + \sum_{i=1}^{n} \sum_{j=1}^{n} \sum_{k=1}^{m} w_{ijk}^2 + \sum_{k=1}^{m} r_k^2$$

In summary, good learning programs work by compressing data. The evaluation of such programs can be done with the minimum-description-length principle, which balances the length of the program against the length of the data when encoded by the program. Since biological programs must work online, this data compression translates into a minimum entropy principle. For that reason living organisms are sometimes colloquially referred to as "entropy eaters."

APPENDIX: LAWS OF PROBABILITY

The basis for probability theory begins with the notion of an event. The universal event U is certain to happen. The chance of an event A happening is denoted by a number associated with the event, $P(A)$. These numbers, termed probabilities, obey the following axioms:

1. The probability of an event A is between zero and one:

$0 \leq P(A) \leq 1$

2. The probability of the certain event denoted U is one:

$P(U) = 1$

3. If events A and B are mutually exclusive, then

$P(A \vee B) = P(A) + P(B)$

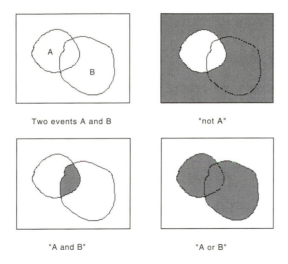

Two events A and B   "not A"

"A and B"   "A or B"

Figure 2.11   The fundamental ideas of probability theory are captured by the Venn diagram, which uses a square denoted U to symbolize the universe of all possible events. Individual events can be described in terms of the event space they take up, denoted in the Venn diagram as a shaded area.

The last axiom uses the symbol $\vee$ for "or." The other standard connectives are $\wedge$ for "and" and $\neg$ for "not." (To remember the difference between $\wedge$ and $\vee$, remember that the $\wedge$ is most like the capital letter A in "And.")

Probabilistic relationships are conveniently visualized using *Venn diagrams,* which use area to denote probability, as shown in Figure 2.11.

Notationally we often write $P(A \wedge B)$ as $P(A, B)$. It follows that

$$P(A) = P(A, B) + P(A, \neg B)$$

$$P(A) + P(\neg A) = 1$$

and

$$P(A) = \sum_{i=1}^{n} P(A, B_i)$$

where the B_i are a set of mutually exclusive events.

In order to use probabilities, there must be a way of interconnecting the way a probability of one event depends on another. This is captured by the notion of the *conditional probability* of A given that B has occurred, written as $P(A \mid B)$.

If A and B are *independent,* then the conditional probability is given by

$$P(A \mid B) = P(A)$$

The *conditional independence* of two events A and B given a third event C is defined as

$$P(A, B \mid C) = P(A \mid C)P(B \mid C)$$

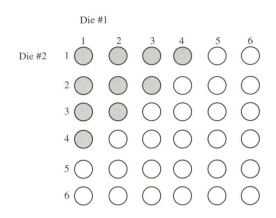

Die #1

Die #2

Figure 2.12   A single roll of two dice. The shaded area of the event space denotes the event "The sum of the two dice is five or less."

Example   Given two dice, what is the probability that their sum is five or less? This question can be answered by computing the following ratio:

$$\frac{\text{Number of throws that add to 5 or less}}{\text{Total number of different throws}}$$

which is 10/36, or 5/18. This result can also be appreciated using a Venn diagram, as shown in Figure 2.12.

NOTES

1. From the introduction to *From Neuron to Brain: A Cellular and Molecular Approach to the Function of the Nervous System,* 3rd ed., by John G. Nicholls, A. Robert Martin, and Bruce G. Wallace (Sunderland, MA: Sinauer, 1992).

2. Zh. I. Reznikova and B. Ya. Ryabko, "Analysis of the Language of Ants by Information-Theoretical Methods," *Problems of Information Transmission* 22, no. 3 (1986):245–49.

3. Another example is the Dempster-Shafer probabilistic inference rule. Ronald R. Yager et al., *Advances in the Dempster-Shafer Theory of Evidence* (New York: Wiley, 1994).

4. Judea Pearl, *Probabilistic Reasoning in Intelligent Systems: Networks of Plausible Inference* (San Mateo, CA: Morgan Kaufmann, 1988).

5. This development follows that of Lassi Hyvärinen in *Information Theory for Systems Engineers* (New York: Springer-Verlag, 1970).

6. Horace B. Barlow, "Single Units and Sensation: A Neuron Doctrine for Perceptual Psychology?" *Perception* 1 (1972):371–94.

7. The examples in this section were drawn from Hyvärinen, *Information Theory,* which also covers the cases of a noisy channel and of error checking.

8. Huffman coding is named after its inventor, David Huffman.

9. John G. Daugman, "High Confidence Visual Recognition of Persons by a Test of Statistical Independence," *Pattern Analysis and Machine Intelligence* 15, no. 11 (November 1993):1148–61.

10. The minimum-description-length principle was introduced by Jorma Rissanen in *Stochastic Complexity in Statistical Inquiry* (Teaneck, NJ: World Scientific, 1989), Chapter 3.

11. The tricky assumption in this analysis is hidden in $P(M)$. Can one really estimate the probability distribution of possible models? This question is what distinguishes "Bayesian" theorists. They think that this is a plausible thing to do. See also Richard S. Zemel in "A Minimum Description Length Framework for Unsupervised Learning" (Ph.D. thesis, Computer Science Department, University of Toronto, 1993).

EXERCISES

1. Use Venn diagrams to show the following events:

a. $(\neg A) \wedge B$
b. $(\neg B) \vee A$
c. $(\neg A) \vee (\neg B)$

2. Use Venn diagrams to prove *de Morgan's laws*:

a. $\neg(A \vee B) = \neg A \wedge \neg B$
b. $\neg(A \wedge B) = \neg A \vee \neg B$

3. Consider a random variable x with mean m and variance σ. Now suppose that you have another independent variable y that is distributed in the same manner. What are the mean and variance of $w = x + y$?

a. Generalize your result for n identically distributed variables.
b. Compute the mean and variance for the sum $w = \Sigma_{i=1}^{n} x_i$ where each $x_i = \pm 1$ with equal probability.

4. Show that the factor $P(D)$ can be regarded as unimportant, as it can always be computed by normalizing.

5. Verify that

$$P(A) = \frac{O(A)}{1 + O(A)}$$

given the definition of $O(A)$.

6. Assume a burglar alarm can be tested so that

$P(Alarm \mid Burglary) = 0.95$

Furthermore we know that the possibility of it going off accidentally is small:

$P(Alarm \mid \neg Burglary) = 0.01$

Assume also that statistics show that $P(Burglary) = 10^{-4}$. In the night the alarm goes off. What is the probability of a burglary given this data?

7. Robbie the Robot's job is to pick up boxes and take them to a designated location, as in the text example. Given the figures from that example, what is the improvement in performance one could realize from two cameras instead of one?

8. For the binomial distribution, show that $E(X) = np$ and $D^2(X/n) = pq/n$.

9. Regarding the problem of the robot camera system, show that

$$P('B' \mid B) + P(\neg 'B' \mid B) = 1$$

but that in general

$$P('B' \mid B) + P('B' \mid \neg B) \neq 1$$

10. On a freeway the average number of passengers in a car is 1.3. What is the probability of having at least two passengers in a randomly selected car? Assume a Poisson process.

11. The equation for *a posteriori* odds can be generalized for multiple sources of evidence $e^1, e^2, \ldots, e^n$. Start with

$$O(H \mid e^1, e^2, \ldots, e^n) = L(e^1, e^2, \ldots, e^n \mid H)O(H)$$

and use conditional independence to simplify this equation. Recall that A and B are conditionally independent, given C if $P(A, B \mid C) = P(A \mid C)P(B \mid C)$. Show also that this formula can be calculated incrementally as new evidence is found, that is, that

$$O(H \mid e^{n+1}) = O(H \mid e^n)L(e^k \mid H)$$

12. During the 1960s computer programs used to be stored on punched cards, on which patterns of holes indicated ASCII symbols. Sixty-four symbols were used, and up to 80 could be stored on one card. Estimate the volume of cards required to represent all possible 80-character messages, given that a box of 2,000 cards takes up 7 liters of space.

13. Consider a problem in tactile sensing in which a stimulus is signaled by its position in an $n \times n$ two-dimensional grid, as shown in Figure 2.13.

a. How many bits are needed to represent the code?
b. What is its information content?

Now consider an alternate strategy of representing the signals with three overlapping sensory grids of $(n/3)^2$ sensors each that are offset from each other by one unit, as shown in the second part of the figure.

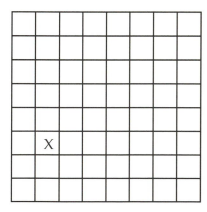
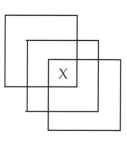

Figure 2.13 Different coding strategies for tactile signaling.

Table 2.5 Code used by the Willy Wonka Chocolate Factory.

Data Block	Code
00	0
01	10
10	110
11	111

c. How many bits are needed to represent the code?

d. What is its information content?

e. What is the savings of the second strategy over the first?

f. What advantage does the original strategy have over this strategy?

Generalize this result to a k-dimensional sensory array.

14. Find a more compact encoding strategy for the tactile array than the one in the previous problem.

15. At the Willy Wonka Chocolate Factory they are constantly making chocolate bars. The computer in charge of the process codes good bars as a zero. Once in a while the machine makes an error, which the computer records as a one. Studies show that the probability of a mistake $P(1) = \frac{1}{16}$, so that $P(0) = \frac{15}{16}$. A sample record is given by

000010000101000000100

a. Based on the probabilities given, what is the information rate or entropy?

b. These data are taking up a lot of space. As a newly employed systems analyst, you suggest that the company encode the data in blocks of two bits using the code shown in Table 2.5. Use the code in the table on the given data stream.

c. What is the minimum number of bits it should take to encode the data stream given in the example?

d. Suggest a better code, and show that it works.

3 Programs

ABSTRACT   A central facet of natural computation is describing its key elements. These are programs. Programs work by searching a *state space* using *operators* that govern the transitions from one state to another. Problem solving can be seen as choosing a good sequence of operators in order to specify a path through state space. *Heuristic search* uses a fitness function to choose between global alternative paths. *Minimax,* for game playing, uses a fitness function to rate local alternative paths.

3.1   INTRODUCTION

The Turing machine model introduced in Chapter 1 captures the basics of a program. The machine has states and arcs (which we will call *operators* here) that specify how to get from one state to another. The collection of states is known as the *state space* of the system. Figure 3.1 shows two such examples. In the first, the state space of three neurons can be represented as a point in a "box" that circumscribes their possible firing rates. Any possible set of firing rates translates to a point in this box. One might conceptualize this state space as continuous, but any real-world signal, such as a firing rate, can always be represented with a discrete number. The reason is fundamental: The real world contains *noise* that corrupts measurements with the result that there is always a limit beyond which further precision in measurements is uninformative. Thus there will be some integer n that captures the useful precision in firing rates. Therefore the number of useful states in the three-neuron system is n^3. If 1,000 were the scaled maximum firing rate, an example of the state of the system would be a list of three firing rates (305, 556, 100). The second example is the two-person game of ticktacktoe. One player uses an X symbol, the other an O symbol. Players alternate turns writing their symbol in a space on a 3×3 grid. The objective is to be the first to complete a line of three in a row. In this system each of the nine squares can have any of three symbols, an X, an O, or a blank, so the number of states is 3^9. Here an example of the state of the system would be a list of the symbols occupying each square. Where b = "blank," such an example would be the list (O, b, b, X, X, O, O, b, X). From these two examples you can see that the state captures the essential degrees of freedom of a system but that there needs to be an additional structure to interpret the state values. In animals, this structure is embodied in the organism itself.

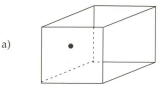

a)

b)

O | |
X | X | O
O | | X

Figure 3.1 Two examples of state spaces. (*a*) A system of three neurons that each have a firing rate that varies from zero spikes/second to 1,000 spikes/second. In this case the "state" of the system can be represented as a point with three associated coordinates each encoding the value of a firing rate. (*b*) The ticktacktoe problem where players alternate turns, each trying to win by making a line of three. In this case the state of the system is a particular board configuration of Xs, Os, or blank squares.

Getting the amount of state to be just right is a huge problem that we will start to address at the end of this chapter. To see that this might be a problem, consider the output of the retina, which has about one million measurements. If the problem is to detect motion, then at any instant only the subset of measurements that are changing are informative, so the state space is too large. On the other hand, if an object is out of view, then all the measurements are uninformative, so the state space is too small. Nonetheless, there are cases where the state can be successfully estimated. Figure 3.2 shows one such case, in which neural responses of cells in the rat have been interpreted as indicating a location in space.[1]

Now let's take up the notion of *operators*. At any point in time you can be "at" a point in state space, and the notion of "at" is captured by the list of essential parameters. Operators specify how to move through a state space. A state space is examined or *searched* incrementally by going to new states and operators govern the transition to a new state from the current state. Figure 3.3 illustrates operators for the two state-space examples. Operators typically have a *Markov* property: They only need a description of the current state to generate the possible successor states. In the case of the neurons, if we denote the combined firing rates by x, then the next state is generated by a function that describes the interactions between neurons, which can be written as a *differential equation*:

$$\frac{dx}{dt} = F(x,u)$$

In this equation u represents parameters of the system, which for the neuron are representations of synapses. The problem is to choose a setting for

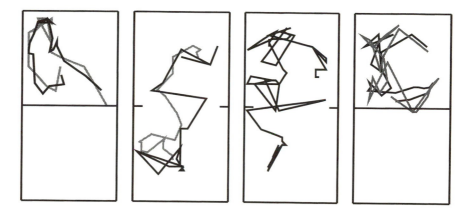

Figure 3.2 Calculating the position of a rat based on direct recordings of neural firing during four transits of a maze. (*black*) Actual positions of rat during maze exploration. (*gray*) Recordings from rat hippocampal cells interpreted as two-dimensional position. (From Wilson and McNaughton, 1993; reprinted with permission from *Science*, © 1993 American Association for the Advancement of Science.)

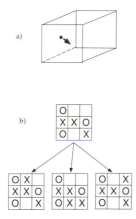

Figure 3.3 Two examples of operators. (*a*) The system of three neurons will have its firing changed according to some function of each neuron's input. The result is that the state will move along a trajectory determined by this dynamics. (*b*) From the ticktacktoe state shown the next player has the X symbol. There are three possible successor states corresponding to the possible places for the X.

u that causes the trajectory of **x** to move in a desired way. In the case of the ticktacktoe example, there are three operators from the state shown corresponding to the three remaining places to put an X. The problem is to try to pick the best of these possibilities from the standpoint of that player's winning chances.

As these examples suggest, the ubiquitous computation that needs to be done is to choose the best of alternative trajectories in state space in a systematic way. Such methods are described as *weak search* methods and can

Three cannibals and three missionaries are on the left bank of a river and want to cross to the opposite bank. They can use a boat that holds two people. If on either bank or in the boat the cannibals outnumber the missionaries, the missionaries will be eaten. The problem is to pick a strategy that gets all of the parties to the opposite side safely.

be characterized by different strategies for exploration of the state space using operators. Two of the most common are *heuristic search* and *minimax*. Heuristic search estimates costs of different paths from an initial state to a goal state. Minimax estimates costs of paths from a current state; it is used in two-person games.

Picking good encodings for a problem's state spaces and operators typically requires ingenuity even when the problem is well specified. To convey the idea of the kinds of choices to be made, consider the classic "cannibals and missionaries" problem (see Box 3.1). You might like to try and solve this problem yourself before seeing the answer.

The first step in setting up the solution is to choose the problem state space. What gets represented? Obviously the names of the cannibals and missionaries are not important. Nor is the color of the boat, the clothes, the people's heights, and so on. Their weight might be relevant in any practical instance of the problem, but since it is not mentioned, assume it is not important. The essence of the problem is just the ratio of cannibals to missionaries at each location. As long as wherever there are missionaries this ratio is less than or equal to unity, no one is eaten. The final step in defining the state space is to divide up the timescale. Again we choose a discrete representation. Consider three different cases: the empty boat at the right bank, the empty boat at the left bank, and the boat loaded in transit.

This important and vital step of defining the discrete state space, which has been done here in an *ad hoc* manner, is the essence of defining a problem, because it is always right to discretize any arbitrary description, even one specified in terms of continuous parameters.

The next step in the specification of the problem solution is to define the operators that allow the transition from one state to another. In this case an operator is simply the number of cannibals and missionaries that end up in the boat. Where (c, m) denotes c cannibals and m missionaries, this can be $(0, 1)$, $(1, 0)$, $(2, 0)$, $(0, 2)$ or $(1, 1)$. As the ferrying process is under way, some operators will not be applicable. For example, if there are no cannibals on a bank, then $(2, 0)$ cannot be used.

Defining the states and operators completes the formulation of the problem. A portion of the state space is shown in Figure 3.4. Now it is just a matter of systematically trying out all the different possibilities. One of the solutions to the problem is shown in Figure 3.5.

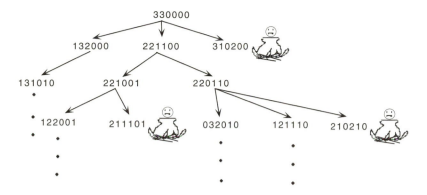

Figure 3.4 Partial specification of the state space for the cannibals and missionaries problem.

L. Bank	Boat	R. Bank	
3:3	0:0	0:0	
1:3	0:2	0:0	Two cannibals get in the boat
1:3	1:0	1:0	One gets left; the other goes back
1:2	1:1	1:0	A cannibal takes a missionary
1:2	1:0	1:1	And leaves him there
1:1	1:1	1:1	The cannibal takes another missionary
1:1	1:0	1:2	And leaves her there
0:1	1:1	1:2	The cannibal takes another cannibal
0:1	1:0	2:2	And leaves him there
0:0	1:1	2:2	The cannibal takes another missionary
0:0	0:0	3:3	Everyone is on the opposite side

Figure 3.5 Steps in the solution of the cannibals and missionaries problem. The state space consists of the number of each on the two banks and in the boat. Operators dictate who gets in the boat.

3.2 HEURISTIC SEARCH

The cannibals and missionaries problem illustrates the core problem with search: The alternatives are not immediately available but are accessed sequentially with operators. The next issue to settle is that of managing the different choices in the search process in a systematic way. The key idea is the use of a *heuristic function* that rates the value of different states according to how far they are from a goal state. This allows the search for a path in state space to be concentrated on states that receive the best ratings by the heuristic function.

Let us formalize this problem in terms of a classical puzzle that carries with it a lot of intuition on the structure of searching.[2] The puzzle is to arrange tiles in a grid to form a pattern. A blank space allows tiles immediately adjacent to the blank to be moved. The size of the grid could be arbitrary, but for simplicity we will study moving eight tiles on a 3 × 3 grid.

3.2.1 The Eight-Puzzle

Formally the problem is to rearrange the eight tiles that are in an *initial state* to form a particular *goal state*. Instinctively we like to put them in numerical order, but the goal state could be any arrangement. For example, consider the problem shown in Figure 3.6.

Here the operators change the tile positions. Describing tile motions could be done by specifying a tile and its possibilities, but a cleverer way is to think of moving the blank (even though that's not what physically happens). Figure 3.7 shows this convention. The possible operators are UP, DOWN, LEFT, and RIGHT. To simplify matters, the option of applying the inverse operator—for example, an UP immediately after a DOWN—is ruled out.

Figure 3.7 is a concrete example of the basic structure for keeping track of the options available in a search: a *tree*. As shown in Figure 3.8, a tree has a *root node*, *internal nodes*, and *leaves*, or *terminal nodes*. By convention the root is at the top and the leaves at the bottom. The nodes immediately below any node are that node's *children*. The node immediately above a node is its *parent*. If there is a route from a node to another that is above it, the latter node is an *ancestor*.

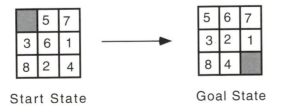

Start State   Goal State

Figure 3.6 An eight-puzzle problem. Starting from the configuration on the left, the objective is to reorder the tiles so as to produce the configuration on the right.

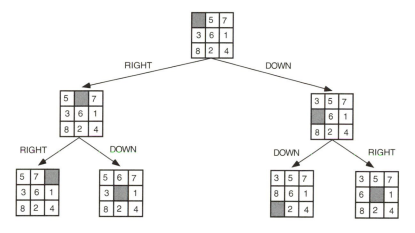

Figure 3.7 Thinking of moving the blank provides a description of the possible operators: LEFT, RIGHT, UP, and DOWN.

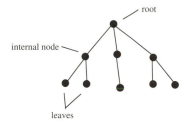

Figure 3.8 Enumerating the possibilities in a search results in a tree. The start node is known as the root of the tree. The nodes accessible from the root are its children. The lower boundary of the tree consists of leaf nodes.

The tree structure is a way of keeping track of the enumeration of the possibilities, but it does not specify any particular order for doing so. Let's consider the various options. The most inexpensive way would be to have a way of rating the choices at a particular node, and then to pick the best at every stage. This method is known as hill climbing or gradient following. It works well if the rating function has a simple structure, such as a single hill. But when the evaluation function is complicated, with many different local maxima, it's easy to get stuck. Sometimes a local maximum is enough, but for the eight-puzzle it means stopping short of the goal.

Another way is to enumerate the nodes in some order. Two systematic ways of doing so are called depth-first and breadth-first. Depth-first search always expands the leftmost (say) node of each successor. If there are none, then the sibling to the right is next, and if all the siblings have been examined, then the parent node is searched for its leftmost unexpanded node. Breadth-first search expands all the nodes at one level before examining nodes at a deeper level. Both these algorithms are easy to formalize, as is done in Algorithm 3.1 for depth-first search. To change depth-first search to breadth-first search, put the expanded nodes at the

Algorithm 3.1 Depth-First Search

1. Examine the start node to see if it is the goal. If so, stop; otherwise expand its successors and, if they do not exceed a *depth bound*, put them on the front of a list called OPEN.

2. If OPEN is empty, then stop with failure.

3. Take the first member of OPEN and examine it to see if it is the goal or if it is on the CLOSED list. If so, stop; otherwise put it on a list called CLOSED, expand it, and put its successors on OPEN.

Algorithm 3.2 Heuristic Search

1. Examine the start node to see if it is the goal. If so, stop; otherwise expand its successors and put them on a list called OPEN.

2. If OPEN is empty, then stop with failure.

3. Take the least-cost member of OPEN and examine it to see if it is the goal. If so, stop; otherwise put it on a list called CLOSED, expand it, and put its successors on OPEN.

back of OPEN instead of the front. Also, you need not worry about the depth bound.

At this point the reader may be thinking that there must be a more informed way of doing this, and there is: *heuristic search.* The idea is to have an evaluation function that rates each of the nodes. Then at each point the best node is selected for expansion. Suppose the function is a cost function. In that case the minimum cost node is selected. The transformation of the earlier algorithm is straightforward (see Algorithm 3.2).

If you think about it, you will realize that the list OPEN contains the frontier of the tree. At any moment the best node in the frontier is selected, and the frontier is expanded at that point. It turns out that the cost function should estimate the cost of the path from the start to the goal. Suppose the search has proceeded to a node n that is in the middle of the search tree, as shown in Figure 3.9. The cost estimate has two parts: the cost from the start to n, and the estimated cost from n to the goal. Thus

$$f(n) = g(n) + h(n)$$

In the eight-puzzle problem a natural cost is the number of moves. Thus

$g(n) = $ Number of moves to get to node n, and

$h(n) = $ Estimated number of moves to get from n to the goal

Now $g(n)$ is known, since it can be counted for each node as the search progresses. The choice of $h(n)$ is more difficult. A function that works is

$h(n) = $ Number of misplaced tiles left at node n

This $h(n)$ underestimates the cost to the goal, since at least one move is necessary to put each tile in place. It turns out that underestimating is crucial

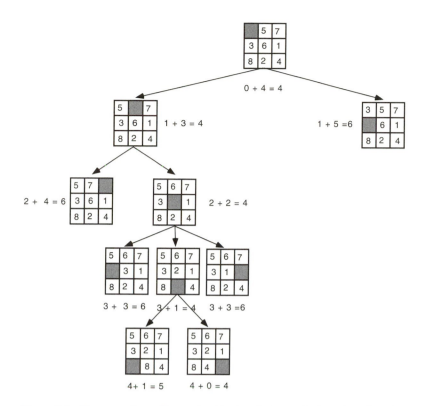

Figure 3.9 The example problem solved by heuristic search. At each node n the crucial information is an estimate of the cost of the current path.

to guarantee that the optimal path is found. This point is easy to see: If $h(n)$ overestimated the cost, then when the goal node was encountered, there might be another path remaining to be discovered that is actually cheaper. With underestimation this difficulty does not arise. If there were a cheaper node, it would already have been encountered. Figure 3.9 shows the result of using the heuristic function to solve the sample problem of Figure 3.6. Using heuristic search, only nine nodes had to be examined. In contrast, a depth-first expansion of the tree would examine 18 nodes before finding the goal.

3.3 TWO-PERSON GAMES

In contrast, two-person games are characterized by considering an adversary's options (moves) in addition to your own. The model we will use works for games of perfect information, such as checkers, chess, backgammon, and Othello, where each side has a complete picture of the game situation. Games of incomplete information, such as poker, bridge, and Stratego, require that decisions be made without complete knowledge of the opponent's holdings. These have to be handled probabilistically.

The moves in a two-person game can be represented as a tree, as shown in Figure 3.10. In this tree, all the moves at each level correspond to the options of one player or the other. The complete set of options whereby two players each have a turn is known as a *ply*. Exhaustively searching 6-ply means looking at all the moves up to 12 moves ahead of the current position.

A crucial difference between heuristic search and game-tree search is that the latter must handle cases where the tree cannot be searched in its entirety. Chess has 10^{120} moves! In this case, game-tree search must look ahead a certain amount (ply) and then choose a move based on that information.

3.3.1 Minimax

Since the game tree cannot be exhaustively searched, the best one can hope for is to make a local decision based on limited look-ahead (Figure 3.11). The look-ahead strategy will expand the tree a fixed number of plies and then score the board positions at the leaf nodes. To do so an evaluation function must be picked that scores different features of the board. Some board positions are easy to rank, such as those in checkers when you are

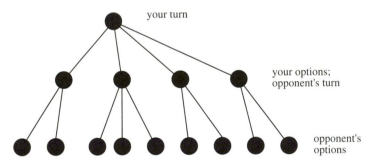

Figure 3.10   A single ply of a hypothetical search tree for a two-person game to illustrate the enumeration of moves. "Your" perspective is shown. All your possible moves form nodes at the first level in a tree. From each of these, enumeration of your opponent's moves results in a subtree.

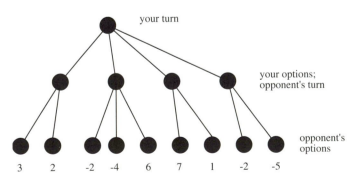

Figure 3.11   The single ply of the hypothetical search tree for a two-person game to illustrate the minimax principle. The numbers at the leaf nodes denote the scores for that position from your point of view.

ahead on pieces, but others are more subtle. Like the function *h* in heuristic search, picking the components of the evaluation function is an art. But suppose that these choices have been made and the results are as shown in the figure. The scores reflect "your" viewpoint. Moves that are good receive positive scores, whereas moves that are bad—that is, good for your opponent—receive negative scores.

The *minimax* procedure (see Algorithm 3.3) allows the evaluations at the tree extremities to be propagated backward to choose your move. Consider the penultimate nodes from left to right. The first choices are two moves with scores of 3 and 2. Your opponent likes negative scores; thus the best move from his or her point of view has a value of 2. Applying this evaluation perspective to the other nodes at this level results in scores of −4, 1, and −5, respectively. Now consider your move, to be planned from the root node. The choices that you have lead to evaluations of 2, −4, 1, and −5. Naturally you are trying to do the best you can, so you pick the move that leads to a score of 2. Hence the name *minimax:* at levels in the tree that represent your moves, you pick the maximum of the scores; at levels that represent your opponent's moves, you pick the minimum of the scores. In this example, the best move is indicated by the leftmost option. You make this move, wait for your opponent's response, and repeat the procedure.

Example: Othello Othello is a two-person game played on an 8×8 board. The pieces are black-and-white disks (black on one side and white on the other). A move consists of placing a disk of your color on an unoccupied square that adjoins a square occupied by your opponent's disk. There must be another disk of your color on a square such that that piece and the played piece straddle a contiguous group of your opponent's disks. The straddled disks then change color. Examples of possible moves are shown in Figure 3.12.

Algorithm 3.3 Minimax

---

1. Set OPEN to be the list of the root of the game tree, *r*.

2. *n* = the first node on OPEN.

3. If *n* = *r* and *n* has a score, then DONE.

4. If *n* has a score, delete *n* from OPEN.

5. If *n* does not have a score and it is a leaf node, then score the game position and assign it to *n*.

6. If *n* has not been scored but all its children have, then

a. If *n* is a maximizing node, set its score to the maximum of its children's scores.

b. If *n* is a minimizing node, set its score to the minimum of its children's scores.

7. If neither *n* nor its children have scores, add the children to the front of OPEN.

8. Go to step 2.

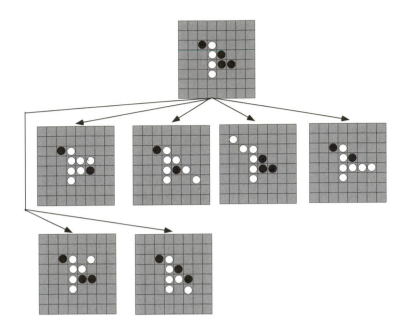

Figure 3.12 A half ply of the search tree for Othello. Six possible moves for white are shown.

3.3.2 Alpha and Beta Cutoffs

The minimax procedure is straightforward and elegant, but it turns out that this is not the best we can do. For example, in the search tree of Figure 3.11, we find that we never have to look at nodes −4, 6, and −5. Why? Remember that your nodes are *maximizing nodes*; the opponent's are *minimizing nodes*. When we have determined that we have searched exhaustively below the leftmost node under the top, that value can be "backed up" to the top as provisional. In fact, let's call it the *provisional backed-up value,* or PBV. In the example, the value of 2 can be provisionally backed up to the root node. Now it is rather obvious that in the course of comparing positions, the value of a maximizing node can only go up and the value of a minimizing node can only go down. Continuing with the example, look at what happens when −2 is encountered. This can be backed up to the minimizing node as its PBV. But above that node you already have an option with a score of 2. There is no point in searching below the minimizing node further, as the score will only go down, and there is already a better option. Generalizing from this example leads to constraints for eliminating possibilities at maximizing and minimizing nodes, called α and β cutoffs, respectively.

1. The PBV of a maximizing node can only increase; thus if a minimizing node below it has a lower value, then search below the minimizing node can be terminated.

2. The PBV of a minimizing node can only decrease; thus if a maximizing node below it has a higher value, then search below the maximizing node can be terminated.

3.4 BIOLOGICAL STATE SPACES

You have no doubt noticed that in introducing state spaces we talked about states at the neural level, as in the three-neuron example, and states at the problem-solving level, as in the ticktacktoe example. Of course, the ultimate goal is to relate these two different levels. We would like to know how neural state spaces represent problem state spaces. There are really two parts to this question. The harder part is to understand the actual solution to this knotty problem. That is the goal of the natural computation enterprise, and its solution is not currently known. The easier part is to understand some crucial issues that the picture of state spaces painted here needs to grapple with. These issues will be tackled in later chapters, but it is useful to highlight them here, as you have probably already started to think of them.

When thinking about the operators that make up the brain's programs, you can think of the repertoire as the set of instructions that can be used. Thus it is conceptually possible to search for a program by trying out the set of instructions that are possible in its state space. Similarly, when thinking about behaviors, you can think of a state space of actions such as picking something up, putting it down, opening it, and so on. Thus it is also possible to search the set of possible actions for a behavior that will accomplish a goal. Therefore, the problem can be rephrased as a search for a representation that relates the neural states of the brain's instruction language to states representing useful properties of the world. In this scenario, the main bugaboos are the uncertainty of the world and the need to describe problem spaces economically. Since the world is uncertain, no matter how an action is described, all its possible effects are very difficult to characterize.[3]

The main method of handling these problems is that of *hidden Markov models.* Such models simultaneously grapple with both of the problems. The fact that the brain states cannot represent all of the aspects of states in the world is explicitly acknowledged by the notion of "hiddenness." What goes on in the world may be hidden from the internal representation. Thus one attempts to characterize the fit between the internal model of the world and the observations from the world probabilistically. The fact that actions can have unpredictable consequences is captured by the "Markovian" assumption that explicitly models actions as having probabilistic effects. The Markovian assumption also comes with the tenet that the current state representation is all that is needed to describe what could happen, albeit probabilistically. All this comes later, in Chapters 10 and 11; however, in order to understand how to handle a probabilistic state space, it helps enormously to have a firm grounding in how to handle a deterministic state space, and that is what this chapter has been about.

NOTES

1. M. A. Wilson and B. L. McNaughton,"Dynamics of the Hippocampal Ensemble Code for Space," *Science* 261 (1993):1055.

2. Introduced by Nils Nilsson in *Problem-Solving Methods in Artificial Intelligence* (New York: McGraw-Hill, 1971).

3. One approach is to attempt to describe what happens in logic. The attraction of this tack is that logical inference can also be characterized as a state-space search. If this enterprise were successful, then problem solving could be mechanized by translating the representation of the world into a logical formalism. In such a formalism, asking whether a problem can be solved is equivalent to proving that its solution (expressed in logic) is a consequence of the axioms that express the description of the problem. Such an enterprise has been the subject of 40 years of intensive research. In addition to classic texts by Winston, Tanimoto, and Rich and Knight, there are two new texts by Dean, Allen, and Aloimonos and by Russell and Norvig: Patrick Henry Winston, *Artificial Intelligence*, 2nd ed. (Reading, MA: Addison-Wesley, 1984); Steven L. Tanimoto, *The Elements of Artificial Intelligence: An Introduction using LISP* (Rockville, MD: Computer Science Press, 1987); Elaine Rich and Kevin Knight, *Artificial Intelligence*, 2nd ed. (New York: McGraw-Hill, 1991); Thomas L. Dean, James F. Allen, and Yiannis Aloimonos, *Artificial Intelligence: Theory and Practice* (Redwood City, CA: Benjamin Cummings, 1995); and Stuart J. Russell and Peter Norvig, *Artificial Intelligence: A Modern Approach* (Englewood Cliffs, NJ: Prentice Hall, 1995). The main problem is to tame the effects of the world by constraining the things that can happen into useful, discrete categories. This paradigm is sometimes seen as being at odds with the natural computation paradigm, but the explanation is more likely just that the problems are defined at a more abstract level of abstraction. Harkening back to Newell's organization of behavior into different timescales (Table 1.3), the suggestion is that logical inference operates at the 10-second timescale whereas the focal timescales of this text extend to the 100-millisecond and one-second scales.

EXERCISES

1. A *topographic map* shows the height of land as a function of a map coordinate $H(x, y)$. Assume that you have a *digitized version $H[i, j]$, $i, j = 1,..., N$* of the map shown in Figure 3.13. Assume that adjacent map locations that differ by more than a certain height d_o are impassable.

a. Describe how you would search for the best path from A to B.
b. What is your heuristic function $f = g + h$?
c. Is your h a lower bound on the optimal h?

2. Given the game-move tree shown in Figure 3.14 from the maximizer's point of view, compute the value of the tree, show the best move, and identify any a or β cutoffs as such.

3. Specify a good evaluation function for Othello. How does your function score the positions in Figure 3.12?

4. Two of your friends are having an argument. One suggests that it would be trivial to extend the eight-puzzle code to its three-dimensional version, the 26-puzzle, and the other says that it is impossible. (Don't get bogged down on how to move the space; maybe we'll use a magnet or something.) Settle the issue one way or the other by either (a) showing that it cannot be done or (b) showing that it can be done by defining the new states, opera-

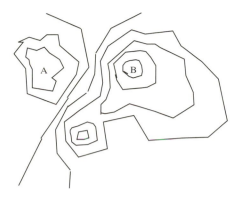

Figure 3.13   Topographic map.

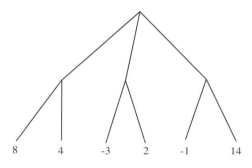

Figure 3.14   Minimax tree.

tors, and heuristic functions. Extend your argument to the *n*-dimensional version of the puzzle.

5. These same two friends are at it again. Now they want to extend the minimax algorithm to the case where one player gets *two* moves for every one taken by the other.

a. Can minimax be extended to handle this case? Explain.

b. Now they are on the same side playing against someone from down the hall. They are using a protocol of alternating moves, first using Marlow's evaluation function for rating the board, and then, on their next turn, using Jonanne's.

i. Can minimax handle this protocol?

ii. Will there be problems in the performance of the system?

6. Consider a three-person game with players ONE, TWO, and THREE. In this game player ONE moves, then TWO, and then THREE. At the leaves of the minimax search tree three numbers are kept for each board position, representing the value of the position from the three players' respective points of view. That is, (3 4 2) means a board position is worth 3 points to player ONE, 4 points to player TWO, and 2 points to player THREE (Figure 3.15). Show how a minimax-like algorithm could handle this case, and demonstrate it on the example.

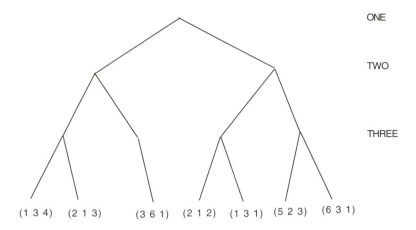

(1 3 4)   (2 1 3)   (3 6 1)   (2 1 2)   (1 3 1) (5 2 3)   (6 3 1)

Figure 3.15   Three-person game tree.

7. Specify an incremental version of the expectation-maximization algorithm in which data are added one point at a time. The idea is to restructure the formulas so as to minimize the calculations after each data point is added.

4 Data

ABSTRACT This chapter introduces the use of a vector to represent a continuous state space. Reducing the size of such state spaces is central to natural computation. One way to reduce their size is to change the dimensionality of the space. Another is to summarize the data in terms of prototype points.

4.1 DATA COMPRESSION

A major part of learning must be triggered just from intrinsic organization in the world. Such organization is reflected in the outputs of our sensors. That output can be described very generally as a set of discrete measurements that have geometric and algebraic properties. The simplest collection of such properties defines a *linear space*. The focus of this chapter is to describe the most basic methods for detecting structure in the state space of such measurements. Its thrust is to develop the basic properties of linear spaces and to show how they can be used to encode collections of data points.

As a motivating problem consider the state space of vision at the output end of the retina, which has about one million independent measurements. These can be recorded in a space of one million *dimensions*. Now suppose you want to make a "fight or flight" decision. This obviously can be represented in a very small dimensional space. Can you choose a much smaller set of dimensions that still captures the useful structure needed to make your decision? It turns out that there are very simple and elegant techniques for approaching this problem. Figure 4.1 shows the two main classes, eigenvectors and clustering. Eigenvector directions point along directions of most variance in the data. In the example, the point p is encoded as a single coordinate and a small residual. Clustering uses a prototype point to encode a group of nearby points. For example, to encode the point p, the coordinates of its prototype are used along with a smaller residual. A savings accrues because the same prototype can be used just once for a group of points. The focus of this chapter will be to describe these techniques.

Eigenspaces assume that the transformation from the higher dimensional space to the lower dimensional space is *linear*. These techniques specify a transformation that preserves the most *variation* in the data. From

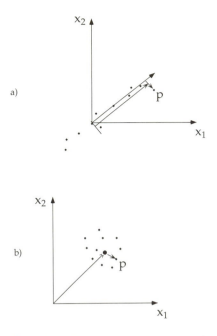

Figure 4.1 The two main classes of techniques for compressing numerical data. (*a*) Eigenvector directions point along directions of most variance in the data. In the example, this technique allows the point *p* to be encoded as a single coordinate and a small residual. (*b*) Clustering uses a prototype point to encode a group of nearby points. In the example, the coordinates of the prototype are sent along with a smaller residual for the point *p*. A savings accrues, since the same prototype can be used for a group of points.

your intuition you might suspect that dimensions along which there is little or no variation other than noise would not be useful at all. As mentioned already, the directions of most variance are the eigenvector directions; the amount of variation along these directions is termed the *eigenvalue*. Eigenvector directions constitute a general coordinate system for state spaces that have enormous usefulness.

Clustering summarizes the distribution of data points in terms of a smaller number of prototype points. A systematic way to compute these prototypes is to guess the number of prototype points and then use the data to adjust the descriptions of their respective probability distributions. A very general way of performing the adjustment is termed *expectation maximization*.[1]

4.2 COORDINATE SYSTEMS

Let us start by considering how coordinate systems represent multi-dimensional data. (If your linear algebra is rusty or fledgling you should scan the appendix to this chapter at this point.) Multiplying a matrix by a vector is a special case of matrix multiplication where

$$y = Ax$$

This can be written as $y_i = \sum_{k=1}^{N} a_{kj} x_j$, $i = 1,\ldots, M$. Alternatively we can see the transformation as a *linear combination* of the columns of A:

$$y = a_1 x_1 + a_2 x_2 + \cdots + a_N x_N$$

Often in manipulating vectors it is implicitly assumed that they are described with respect to an orthogonal coordinate system. Hence the actual coordinate vectors are not discussed. In the general case, however, the right coordinate system for data might not be orthogonal. To develop this point, consider first that the vectors a_i have a special interpretation as a coordinate system or *basis* for a multidimensional space. For example, in the traditional basis in three dimensions,

$$a_1 = \begin{pmatrix} 1 \\ 0 \\ 0 \end{pmatrix}, \ a_2 = \begin{pmatrix} 0 \\ 1 \\ 0 \end{pmatrix}, \text{ and } a_3 = \begin{pmatrix} 0 \\ 0 \\ 1 \end{pmatrix}$$

allows y to be written as

$$y = a_1 y_1 + a_2 y_2 + a_3 y_3$$

A fundamentally important property of coordinate systems is that they are only describable *relative* to one another. For example, y is described in terms of the basis vectors a_i.

This basis is orthogonal, since

$$a_i \cdot a_j = 0$$

for all i and j such that $i \neq j$, but it turns out that a nonorthogonal basis would also work. For example,

$$A = \begin{bmatrix} 1 & 0 & 0 \\ 0 & 1 & 0 \\ -1 & 1 & -1 \end{bmatrix}$$

would still allow y to be represented (although the coefficients would of course be different). However, the matrix

$$A = \begin{bmatrix} 1 & 0 & 0 \\ 0 & 1 & 0 \\ -1 & 1 & 0 \end{bmatrix}$$

would not work. In this case the reason is easy to see: there is no way of representing the third component. In general, to represent n-dimensional vectors, the basis must *span* the space. A general condition for this is that the columns of A must be *linearly independent*. Formally this means that the only way you could write

$$a_1 x_1 + a_2 x_2 + \cdots + a_N x_N = 0$$

would be if $x_i = 0$ for all i.

What happens when the columns of an n-dimensional matrix do not span the space? The dimension of the matrix is equal to the number of linearly independent vectors, which is known as the *rank* of the matrix. When the rank r is less than the dimension N, the vectors are said to span an r-dimensional *subspace*.

In some cases it is desirable for a matrix to have less than full rank. For example, for the equation

$$Ax = 0$$

to have a nontrivial solution, the columns of A must be linearly dependent. Why? This equation is just a rewritten version of the previous equation. If the columns were linearly independent, then the only way the equations could be satisfied would be to have $x_i = 0$ for all i. But for a nontrivial solution the x_i should be nonzero. Hence for this to happen the columns must be linearly *dependent*. For example, in three dimensions this can happen when all three of the vectors are in a plane.

In contrast, for the equation

$$Ax = c$$

to have a unique solution the converse is true, because in order to have a solution, now the vector c must be expressed in terms of a linear combination of the columns a_i. For this statement to be generally true the columns must span the space of c; hence, together with the vector c, they must be linearly dependent. These two cases are illustrated in Figure 4.2.

Coordinate transforms of the form $y = Wx$ can be implemented in a neural network. The way this procedure is done is to define linear neural

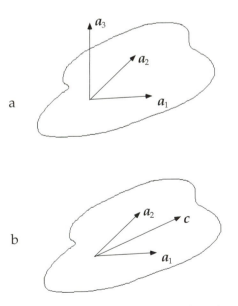

Figure 4.2 (*a*) The columns of A are linearly independent in three dimensions if the three column vectors are not coplanar. (*b*) For the case $Ax = c$ the vector c must lie in the space spanned by A. In two dimensions, therefore, a_1, a_2, and c must all be coplanar.

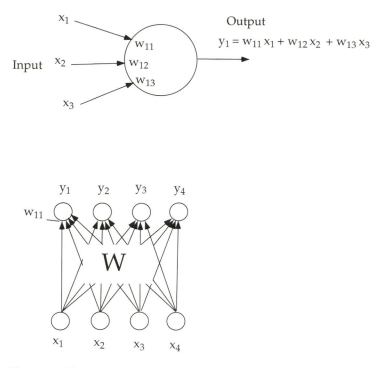

$$y_1 = w_{11} x_1 + w_{12} x_2 + w_{13} x_3$$

Figure 4.3 The basic matrix multiplication used in a linear coordinate transformation can be implemented in a linear neural network.

circuit elements, as shown in Figure 4.3. The basic element has *weights,* or very simple "synapses." (The use of W for the matrix instead of A is just to remind you that the elements are model synapses.) Each weight multiplies with its respective input value. The result of all the pairwise multiplications is then summed as shown in the figure. In the neural network separate units represent the different components of the output vector, as shown.

4.3   EIGENVALUES AND EIGENVECTORS

At this point you should be used to the idea that any matrix can be thought of as representing a coordinate system. When a vector is multiplied by such a matrix, the general result is that the magnitude and direction of the resultant vector are different from the original. However, there is a very important special case. For any matrix, there are vector directions such that the matrix multiplication changes only the magnitude of the vector, leaving the direction unchanged. For these special directions, matrix multiplication reduces to scalar multiplication. The following example shows a case for the matrix

$$\begin{bmatrix} 3 & 1 \\ 2 & 2 \end{bmatrix}$$

where

$$\binom{1}{1}$$

is a special direction for the matrix, since multiplying it by the matrix just results in scaling the vector by a factor $\lambda = 4$; that is,

$$\begin{bmatrix} 3 & 1 \\ 2 & 2 \end{bmatrix} \binom{1}{1} = 4 \binom{1}{1}$$

In the general case, if a vector v lies along one of these directions,

$$Wv = \lambda v$$

where λ is a scalar. Vectors that lie along these special directions are known as *eigenvectors,* and the scalars associated with a transformation matrix are known as *eigenvalues.* Finding the eigenvalues of an $n \times n$ matrix for arbitrary n requires a trip to the recipe book,[2] starting with the solution of an nth-order polynomial to find the eigenvalues, but it is useful to work it out for an easy two-dimensional case, as follows:

$$\begin{bmatrix} 3 & 1 \\ 2 & 2 \end{bmatrix} \binom{v_1}{v_2} = \lambda \binom{v_1}{v_2}$$

or, in other words,

$$\begin{bmatrix} 3 - \lambda & 1 \\ 2 & 2 - \lambda \end{bmatrix} \binom{v_1}{v_2} = \binom{0}{0}$$

From the previous section we know that for this equation to have a solution, the columns of the matrix must be linearly dependent, and thus $|W| = 0$. Thus

$$(3 - \lambda)(2 - \lambda) - 2 = 0$$

which can be solved to find the two eigenvalues $\lambda_1 = 4$ and $\lambda_2 = 1$. Now for the eigenvectors. Substituting $\lambda_1 = 4$ into the equation results in

$$\begin{bmatrix} -1 & 1 \\ 2 & -2 \end{bmatrix} \binom{v_1}{v_2} = \binom{0}{0}$$

Now this set of equations is degenerate, meaning that there is only one useful equation in two unknowns. As a consequence there is an infinity of solutions, and you must pick one arbitrarily. Pick $v_1 = 1$. Then $v_2 = 1$. Thus the eigenvector associated with $\lambda_1 = 4$ is

$$\binom{1}{1}$$

As an easy exercise you can find the eigenvector associated with $\lambda_2 = 1$.

Now, for any particular matrix, why not pick the eigenvectors as the basis? It turns out that this is a good thing to do, since the effect is to transform the matrix into another matrix whose only nonzero elements are on

Chapter 4 Data

the diagonal. Furthermore, these diagonal elements are the eigenvalues. The effect is to reduce matrix multiplication in the old basis to scalar multiplication in the new basis.

To see this point requires understanding the operation of a coordinate transformation. This changes the basis vectors that are representing a vector to another set. A key question is, What happens to transformations when the coordinate basis is changed?

Suppose that the coordinate transformation is given by

$$x^* = Ax$$

$$y^* = Ay$$

Given the transformation

$$y = Wx$$

what happens to W when the coordinate system is changed to the starred system? That is, for some W^* it will be true that

$$y^* = W^*x^*$$

What is the relation between W and W^*? One way to find out is to change back to the original system, transform by W, and then transform back to the starred system; that is,

$$x = A^{-1}x^*$$

$$y = Wx$$

$$y^* = Ay$$

Putting these transformations together:

$$y^* = AWA^{-1}x^*$$

Since the vector transformation taken by the two different routes should be the same, it must be true that

$$W^* = AWA^{-1}$$

Matrices related in this way are called *similar*.

Now let's relate this discussion to eigenvectors. Suppose that the eigenvectors have been chosen as the basis set. Then for a given eigenvector y_i,

$$Wy_i = \lambda y_i$$

and if Y is a matrix whose columns are the eigenvectors y_i, then

$$WY = Y\Lambda$$

Here Λ is a matrix whose only nonzero components are the diagonal elements λ_i. Premultiplying both sides by Y^{-1},

$$Y^{-1}WY = \Lambda$$

What this equation means is that given a matrix W, the transformation it defines can always be simplified to that of a matrix whose only nonzero elements are diagonal by transforming to coordinates that use its eigen-vectors as a basis. Furthermore, those elements are the eigenvalues.

To check this result, let us use the earlier example where

$$W = \begin{bmatrix} 3 & 1 \\ 2 & 2 \end{bmatrix}$$

and

$$Y = \begin{bmatrix} 1 & 1 \\ 1 & -2 \end{bmatrix}$$

and

$$\Lambda = \begin{bmatrix} 4 & 0 \\ 0 & 1 \end{bmatrix}$$

Let us pick a particular vector as x

$$x = \begin{pmatrix} 3 \\ 4 \end{pmatrix}$$

so that y is given by

$$y = \begin{pmatrix} 13 \\ 14 \end{pmatrix}$$

First note that

$$Y^{-1} = \frac{1}{3} \begin{bmatrix} 2 & 1 \\ 1 & -1 \end{bmatrix}$$

so that $x^* = Y^{-1}x$, which is

$$\begin{pmatrix} \frac{10}{3} \\ -\frac{1}{3} \end{pmatrix}$$

and $y^* = Y^{-1}y$, which is

$$\begin{pmatrix} \frac{40}{3} \\ -\frac{1}{3} \end{pmatrix}$$

But from this you can see that $y^* = \Lambda x^*$.

Eigenvalues and eigenvectors have many useful properties, some of which are summarized here (see Box 4.1).

4.3.1 Eigenvalues of Positive Matrices

An important special case occurs when a matrix is positive. Recall that this occurs when $A > 0$. The main consequence is known as the Frobenius-Perron theorem.[3]

Box 4.1   Useful Properties of Eigenvalues and Eigenvectors

> 1. An eigenvalue matrix Λ is invariant under any orthogonal transformation.
>
> 2. If all its eigenvalues are positive, a matrix A is positive definite.
>
> 3. The trace of A is the sum of all its eigenvalues and is invariant under any orthogonal transformation.
>
> 4. The trace of A^m is the sum of all its eigenvalues and is invariant under any orthogonal transformation.
>
> 5. The determinant of A is equal to the product of all its eigenvalues and is invariant under any orthogonal transformation.

Theorem 1 (Frobenius-Perron)   If $A > 0$ then there exists a $\lambda_0 > 0$ and $x_0 > 0$ such that

1. $Ax_0 = \lambda_0 x_0$
2. $\lambda_0 \geq$ any other eigenvalue of A
3. λ_0 is unique

This theorem can also be extended to the case when $A \geq 0$, but there is some n such that $A^n > 0$. In this case all the conclusions of the theorem still apply to A.

It is rather easy to derive bounds on the eigenvalue λ_0. Recall that the eigenvector is only specified up to a scale factor, so that you can normalize it so that $\sum_{i=1}^{n} x_i = 1$. Next expand $Ax_0 = \lambda_0 x_0$ as

$$a_{11}x_1 + a_{12}x_2 + \cdots + a_{1n}x_n = \lambda_0 x_1$$

$$a_{12}x_1 + a_{22}x_2 + \cdots + a_{2n}x_n = \lambda_0 x_2$$

$$\vdots$$

$$a_{n1}x_1 + a_{n2}x_2 + \cdots + a_{nn}x_n = \lambda_0 x_n$$

Now add these equations together to obtain

$$S_{n1}x_1 + S_{n2}x_2 + \cdots + S_{nn}x_n = \lambda_0$$

where $S_1 = a_{11} + a_{21} + \cdots + a_{n1}$, and so on. In other words, the S_i represent the sums of the columns of A. Also, the right-hand-side result uses the fact that the x_i's summed to one. This reasoning leads to the important conclusion that the largest that λ_0 could be is determined by the largest of the S_i's, since the x_i's sum to one, and the maximum value would be achieved if x_i was one for that S_i. Thus λ_0 is bounded by

$$\min_i S_i \leq \lambda_0 \leq \max_i S_i$$

A similar argument can be made for the rows of A. The tighter of these two bounds is the more useful.

4.4 RANDOM VECTORS

Up to this point the matrices have been completely arbitrary. But now let's consider the very important case in which the matrix is defined by variations in a set of data vectors. In this case vectors are drawn from some random distribution that captures the natural variations in the world. A random vector X is specified by a probability density function $p(X)$, where formally

$$p(X) = \lim_{\Delta x_i \to 0} \frac{P(X \in I)}{\prod_i \Delta x_i}$$

where

$$I = \{X : x_i < X_i \le x_i + \Delta x_i , \forall i\}$$

Although a random vector is fully characterized by its density function, such functions are often difficult to determine or mathematically complex to use. These limitations motivate modeling distributions with functions that can be described by a low number of parameters. The most important of such parameters are the *mean vector* and *covariance matrix*, which are just generalizations of the mean and variance of scalar random variables to vector random variables.

The mean vector is defined by

$$M = E\{X\} = \int X p(X) dX$$

and the covariance matrix by

$$\Sigma = E\{(X - M)(X - M)^T\}$$

In practice, with real data you will use the sample mean vector and sample covariance matrix. Where X^k, $k = 1, N$ are the samples,

$$M = \frac{1}{N} \sum_{k=1}^{N} X^k$$

$$\Sigma = \frac{1}{N} \sum_{k=1}^{N} (X^k - M)(X^k - M)^T$$

You will need more than three samples in practice, but to illustrate the calculations, suppose

$$X^1 = \begin{pmatrix} -1 \\ 3 \\ 1 \end{pmatrix}, X^2 = \begin{pmatrix} 2 \\ 1 \\ -1 \end{pmatrix}, X^3 = \begin{pmatrix} 2 \\ 2 \\ 3 \end{pmatrix}$$

Then the mean value is

$$M = \frac{1}{3} \begin{pmatrix} 3 \\ 6 \\ 3 \end{pmatrix} = \begin{pmatrix} 1 \\ 2 \\ 1 \end{pmatrix}$$

So that

$$X^1 - M = \begin{pmatrix} -2 \\ 1 \\ 0 \end{pmatrix}, X^2 - M = \begin{pmatrix} 1 \\ -1 \\ -2 \end{pmatrix}, X^3 - M = \begin{pmatrix} 1 \\ 0 \\ 2 \end{pmatrix}$$

and the covariance matrix is given by

$$\Sigma = \frac{1}{3} \left\{ \begin{bmatrix} 4 & -2 & 0 \\ -2 & 1 & 0 \\ 0 & 0 & 0 \end{bmatrix} + \begin{bmatrix} 1 & -1 & -2 \\ -1 & 1 & 2 \\ -2 & 2 & 4 \end{bmatrix} + \begin{bmatrix} 1 & 0 & 2 \\ 0 & 0 & 0 \\ 2 & 0 & 4 \end{bmatrix} \right\}$$

$$= \frac{1}{3} \begin{bmatrix} 6 & -3 & 0 \\ -3 & 2 & 2 \\ -2 & 2 & 8 \end{bmatrix}$$

Now we can explain why this setting is so important. Consider an arbitrary set of random data vectors sampled from a particular $P(X)$, as shown in Figure 4.4. For any set of coordinate axes, the data will exhibit some variation when projected onto those axes. Suppose the data were clumped in some interesting way. Such clumps can be all-important, as they define natural classes that can be used in decision making. Thus one would like to be able to choose the coordinates to maximally reveal the clumps. It turns out, as will be shown in a moment, that these coordinate directions

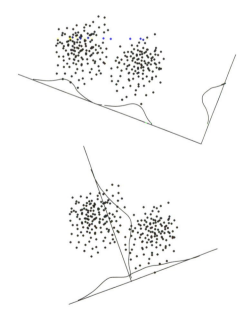

Figure 4.4 Choosing coordinates to maximize the variance can simplify decision making. (*top*) Eigenvector directions result in a distribution along the principal eigenvalue direction that is bimodal, so that two natural classes can be discerned. (*bottom*) Other directions are less likely to reveal such structure.

are the eigenvectors of the covariance matrix. Furthermore, the most important directions, the ones with the most variation, are revealed by having large eigenvalues.

4.4.1 Normal Distribution

As we saw in Chapter 3, one of the most useful parametric distributions is the normal distribution. This statement is true because most observed random variables tend to be the sum of several random components, and the sum of random components tends to be normally distributed. The vector version of the normal distribution, $N(X, M, \Sigma)$, is given by

$$N(X, M, \Sigma) = \frac{e^{-\frac{1}{2}d^2(X, M, \Sigma)}}{2\pi^{-\frac{n}{2}}|\Sigma|^{\frac{1}{2}}}$$

where d^2 is given by

$$d^2(X, M, \Sigma) = (X - M)^T \Sigma^{-1}(X - M)$$

4.4.2 Eigenvalues and Eigenvectors of the Covariance Matrix

In developing the description of a normal distribution, the choice of coordinates has been completely general. Now let's try to pick coordinates that simplify the description of the distribution. In particular, let's pick coordinates that maximize the variance of the distribution. As you can guess, the natural coordinates turn out to be eigenvectors. First transform X to the origin by picking a new random vector Z such that

$$Z = X - M$$

Thus the quadratic form becomes

$$d^2(Z, 0, \Sigma) = Z^T \Sigma^{-1} Z$$

Now let's try to find a Z such that $Z^T Z = 1$ and $d^2(Z, 0, \Sigma)$ is maximized. It turns out that a condition for this to be true is that

$$\Sigma Z = \lambda Z \qquad\qquad\qquad (4.1)$$

In other words, Z must be an eigenvector of the covariance matrix with eigenvalue λ. (It is easy to show this fact, but we need the techniques of the next chapter.)

The principal result can be summarized as follows. Let Φ be an $n \times n$ matrix of the n eigenvectors of Σ. That is,

$$\Phi = [Z_1, Z_2, \cdots, Z_n]$$

Then, summarizing Equation 4.1,

$$\Sigma\Phi = \Phi\Lambda$$

$$\Phi^T\Phi = I$$

where Λ is a diagonal matrix of eigenvalues,

$$\Lambda = \begin{bmatrix} \lambda_1 & \cdots & 0 \\ \vdots & \ddots & \vdots \\ 0 & \cdots & \lambda_n \end{bmatrix}$$

It turns out that a similar result can be arrived at by starting with the constraint that Φ is any orthonormal transformation.

The virtue of the eigenvalues is that they rank the dimensions of the space in terms of variation along those dimensions, and that this ranking is very often related to their importance. In particular, to approximate the variance with the least amount of error using only m dimensions, where $m < n$, simply choose the eigenvectors associated with the m largest eigenvalues. It can be shown that the mean squared error for doing so is simply the sum of the remaining $n - m$ eigenvalues.

Example: A Network That Encodes Data   Earlier you saw that any matrix operation could be realized in a linear neural network. Now let's extend that example to show how a network can encode data. As Figure 4.5a

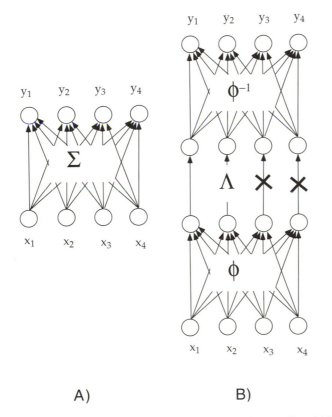

A)   B)

Figure 4.5 Using eigenvector transformations for encoding. (*a*) The covariance matrix can be realized in a network. (*b*) Equivalently, the same transformation can be realized as a succession of three network operations. This formulation allows the data to be encoded (with some error), as the components corresponding to the smallest eigenvalues can be dropped.

shows, a covariance matrix can be represented in terms of network operations. But since multiplication by Σ is equivalent to multiplication by $\Phi\Lambda\Phi^{-1}$, an equivalent network can be built that has three such operations, as shown in Figure 4.5b. This network needs only n connections in the middle owing to the factorization brought about by the eigenvector transformation. Now imagine that the connections with the smallest eigenvalues are dropped as implied by the "X"s. Then the network will approximate or encode the data with an error that is proportional to the sum of the remaining eigenvalues. Note also on the figure that once you remove the connections for the smallest eigenvalues, you don't need the part of the network that was depending on them either, and that can be removed also.

4.5 HIGH-DIMENSIONAL SPACES

All of these operations will be made clear with an example after one more development. Suppose, as is often the case, that the dimension of the space is extremely large. Now the standard way to proceed would be to choose eigenvectors u_k and eigenvalues λ_k of the sample covariance matrix Σ where

$$\Sigma = \frac{1}{M} \sum_{n=1}^{M} X_n X_n^T$$

$$= AA^T$$

where

$$A = [X_1, X_2, \ldots, X_M]$$

an $M \times N$ matrix of M data samples. The problem with this tack is that it is infeasible owing to the high dimensionality of the matrix Σ. Since for an image the dimension of X is n^2, then the dimension of Σ is $n^2 \times n^2$. For typical values of n, say 256, this is impossibly large. Salvation comes from the fact that the matrix Σ may be approximated by a matrix of lower rank. That is, most of the variation can be captured by projecting the data onto a subspace whose dimension is much less than the dimension of the space.

Rather than finding the eigenvectors of the larger system, consider finding the eigenvectors of the $M \times M$ system

$$A^T A v = \mu v \tag{4.2}$$

Premultiplying both sides by A,

$$AA^T A v = \mu A v$$

What this equation shows is that if v is an eigenvector of $A^T A$, then Av is an eigenvector of Σ. Furthermore, the eigenvalues of the smaller system are the same as those of the much larger system. It turns out also that these are the M largest eigenvalues. So to find the eigenvectors of the larger system, first find the eigenvalues and eigenvectors of the smaller system, and then multiply the eigenvectors by A.

Example: Face Recognition A lovely example of representing data is from face recognition.[4] The task is to recognize the identity of an image of a face. The face image is described by an $N \times N$ array of brightness values. Given M exemplars of images with known identities, the objective is to take a new image and identify it with the training image to which it is most similar. The key element is in the similarity metric. It should be chosen to score the essential variations in the data. From the last section, the way to discover the essential variations is with principal components analysis, which identifies the eigenvalues of the covariance matrix of all the data.

To begin, identify the training set of images as $I_1, I_2, \ldots, I_M$. These are shown in Figure 4.6. To work with these it is useful to subtract the bias introduced, as all the brightness levels are positive. Thus first identify the "average face" (shown in Figure 4.7)

$$I_{ave} = \frac{1}{M} \sum_{n=1}^{M} I_n$$

and then convert the training set by subtracting the average,

$$X_i = I_i - I_{ave}, \; i = 1, \ldots, M$$

Now use Equation 4.2 to find M eigenvectors v_k and eigenvalues λ_k.

From the "short" eigenvectors (of length M), the larger eigenvectors u_k, termed eigenfaces, can be constructed using v_k, as follows:

$$u_i = \sum_{k=1}^{M} v_{ik} X_k$$

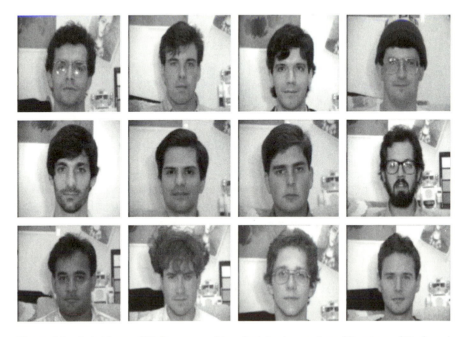

Figure 4.6 A database of 12 figures used to calculate eigenvectors. (Courtesy of Turk and Pentland, 1992.)

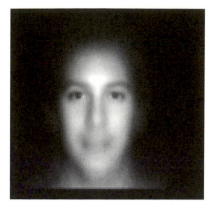

Figure 4.7   The average face (I_{ave}). (Courtesy of Turk and Pentland, 1992.)

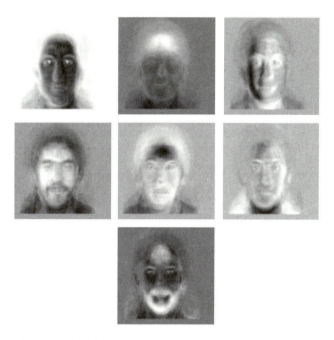

Figure 4.8   The first seven eigenvectors calculated. (Courtesy of Turk and Pentland, 1992.)

Figure 4.8 shows the first seven eigenvectors calculated from Equation 4.2.

Now that the direction principal variations have been calculated in the space of faces, this information can be used to classify a new face in terms of the faces in the data set. To do so, compute the coordinates of the new image in the eigenvector space $\mathbf{\Omega} = (\omega_1, \omega_2, \cdots, \omega_M)$ as follows:

$$\omega_k = \mathbf{u}_k^T (I - I_{ave}), k = 1, \cdots, M$$

Next compare $\mathbf{\Omega}$ to the $\mathbf{\Omega}$s for each of the classes to pick the closest; that is, pick the class k that minimizes

$$\|\mathbf{\Omega} - \mathbf{\Omega}_k\|$$

4.6 CLUSTERING

We now turn to the second method of data compression, that of clustering or prototype points. To see how to make a reduced number of states from "raw" data, consider the case of a set of measurements x_i, $i = 1,\ldots, n$. In that case you could fit them with a Gaussian such that its mean is given by

$$m = \frac{1}{n} \sum_{i=1}^{n} x_i$$

and its variance as

$$\sigma^2 = \frac{1}{n} \sum_{i=1}^{n} (x_i - m)^2$$

The notion is that the measurements are all instances of a single internal state, and the observed deviations can be succinctly described by the mean and variance.

The case of two or more internal states is a little harder but can be handled similarly. The explanation is lengthy but easy to follow given the concepts of the previous chapter. Suppose that the observed data can now be a *mixture* of two states, $k = 1, 2$, and that $P(k)$ is the probability of the kth state.

Let's assume that each of these can be described by a Gaussian; that is,

$$p(x_i \mid k) = \frac{1}{\sqrt{2\pi}\sigma_k} e^{-\frac{(x_i - m_k)^2}{2\sigma_k^2}} \text{ for } k = 1, 2; i = 1,\ldots, n$$

Now the probability of seeing the data sample can be written in terms of the internal state using Bayes' rule:

$$p(x_i) = \sum_{k} p(x_i \mid k) P(k)$$

so that if you are given the data and want to estimate the probability that it came from a particular state you can use Bayes' rule:

$$P(k \mid x_i) = \frac{p(x_i \mid k) P(k)}{\sum_{j} p(x_i \mid j) P(j)} \tag{4.3}$$

This equation in turn allows the *a priori* state probabilities to be estimated as an average

$$P(k) = \frac{1}{n} \sum_{i} P(k \mid x_i) \tag{4.4}$$

Now the probability of seeing all the data, given that the samples are generated independently, is

$$p(x_1,\ldots, x_n) = \prod_{i} \sum_{k} p(x_i \mid k) P(k)$$

Algorithm 4.1   Estimating States with Expectation Maximization

---

Initialize the model by guessing values for m_k and σ_k. Until the model parameters converge, do the following:

1. Choose the internal state probabilistically according to Equation 4.4, which in turn uses Equation 4.3.

2. Now that the state is estimated, update its parameters by using Equation 4.5

$$m_k = \frac{\sum_i P(k \mid x_i) x_i}{\sum_i P(k \mid x_i)}$$

and Equation 4.6

$$\sigma_k = \frac{\sum_i P(k \mid x_i)(x_i - m_k)^2}{\sum_i P(k \mid x_i)}$$

To choose the parameters for each of the internal states, use maximum likelihood estimation by maximizing the log likelihood function given by

$$\log L = \log p(x_1, \ldots, x_n) = \sum_i \log \sum_k p(x_i \mid k) P(k)$$

From calculus you know that at the maximum, the partial derivatives with respect to the parameters will be zero; that is,

$$\frac{\partial \log L}{\partial m_k} = \sum_i p(x_i \mid k) \frac{(x_i - m_k)}{\sigma_k^2} = 0 \tag{4.5}$$

$$\frac{\partial \log L}{\partial \sigma_k^2} = \sum_i p(x_i \mid k) \frac{(x_i - m_k)^2 - \sigma_k^2}{2\sigma_k^4} = 0 \tag{4.6}$$

These equations can be solved for expressions for m_k and σ_k in terms of the data points x_i (see Algorithm 4.1).

APPENDIX: LINEAR ALGEBRA REVIEW

This appendix provides a quick review of the needed concepts from linear algebra, particularly vectors and matrices and their related properties.

Vectors   To begin, let us describe an element of the state space as a point with numerical coordinates, that is

$$x = \begin{pmatrix} x_1 \\ x_2 \\ \vdots \\ x_n \end{pmatrix}$$

These coordinates may be thought of as the components of a *vector*. Vectors of up to three dimensions are easy to diagram. For example,

$$x = \begin{pmatrix} 3 \\ 2 \\ 5 \end{pmatrix}$$

can be drawn as in Figure 4.9.

Addition   To add two vectors together, simply add their components. To multiply a vector by a scalar (number), multiply each of the components by the scalar. For example, if $z = x + y$, then if

$$x = \begin{pmatrix} 3 \\ 5 \\ 2 \end{pmatrix} \quad \text{and} \quad y = \begin{pmatrix} -4 \\ 1 \\ 3 \end{pmatrix} \quad \text{then} \quad z = \begin{pmatrix} -1 \\ 6 \\ 5 \end{pmatrix}$$

And if $z = ax$ for a scalar a, then

$$z = a \begin{pmatrix} 3 \\ 5 \\ 2 \end{pmatrix} = \begin{pmatrix} 3a \\ 5a \\ 2a \end{pmatrix}$$

Dot Product   The *dot product* of two vectors, denoted $x \cdot y$, is defined as the sum of the product of their pairwise components; that is,

$$x \cdot y = \sum_{i=1}^{n} x_i y_i$$

For our example, $x \cdot y = (3)(-4) + (5)(1) + (2)(3) = -1$.

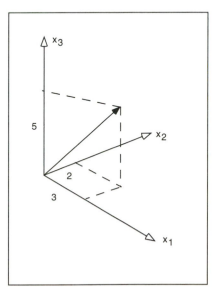

Figure 4.9   An example of a vector.

Appendix: Linear Algebra Review

Two vectors are said to be *orthogonal* if their dot product is zero; that is, $x \cdot y = 0$.

The *length* of a vector, denoted $\|x\|$, is simply $\sqrt{x \cdot x}$. The angle θ between two vectors x and y is given by

$$\cos \theta = \frac{x \cdot y}{\|x\| \, \|y\|}$$

From this equation it is seen that if vectors are orthogonal, then $\cos \theta = 0$ or $\theta = 90°$.

The vector $(x \cdot y)\frac{y}{\|y\|}$ is termed the *projection* of x onto y.

The $\otimes$ Operator   A special operator that will be useful later is $\otimes$, defined for three equal-length vectors x, y, and z, as

$$z = x \otimes y$$

where

$$z_i = x_i y_i, \, i = 1, \ldots, N$$

Matrices   A matrix is an $N \times M$ element array; that is,

$$A = \begin{bmatrix} a_{11} & a_{12} & \cdots & a_{1M} \\ a_{21} & & & \\ \vdots & & & \\ a_{N1} & \cdots & \cdots & a_{NM} \end{bmatrix}$$

Another way to write A is in terms of its elements $\{a_{ij}\}$.

The *transpose* of a matrix, denoted A^T, is simply described using the element notation as $\{a_{ji}\}$. In other words, the elements are "flipped" about the diagonal. A square $n \times n$ matrix is *symmetric* if $A^T = A$.

Linear Transformations   For any function $f(x)$, a linear transformation is such that

$$f(ax + by) = af(x) + bf(y)$$

An important linear transformation is *matrix multiplication*. Matrix multiplication $A = BC$ is defined by

$$a_{ij} = \sum_{k=1}^{N} b_{ik} c_{kj}, \, i = 1, \ldots, P, j = 1, \ldots, Q$$

From this formula it is seen that the number of columns of B has to be the same as the number of rows of C for multiplication to be defined.

Determinant   To define the *determinant* of a matrix first requires defining the number of inversions in a number sequence. Consider the sequence $\{1, 3, 4, 2\}$. The number of inversions in this sequence is 2 because 3 and 4 come after 2. Similarly the number of inversions in {4, 2, 1, 3} is 3. Denote the number of inversions of a sequence as n. The determinant of a matrix A, denoted $|A|$, is the sum of all $n!$ possible different products that compose elements from columns of the matrix with a term that depends on the number of inversions in the row indices; that is,

$$|A| = \sum (-1)^{n(i_1, i_2, \ldots, i_n)} a_{i_1, 1} a_{i_2, 2} \cdots a_{i_n, n}$$

Like the inverse of a matrix, the determinant is expensive to calculate for large matrices, and a standard text should be referred to for an algorithm.[5] For practice calculations, however, it is useful to remember that the determinant of the 2×2 matrix

$$A = \begin{bmatrix} a & b \\ c & d \end{bmatrix}$$

is given by

$$|A| = ad - bc$$

Inverse   For square matrices where $N = M$, an important matrix is the *inverse* matrix A^{-1}, which is defined by

$$AA^{-1} = I$$

where I is the *identity matrix*

$$I = \begin{bmatrix} 1 & 0 & \cdots & 0 \\ 0 & 1 & & \vdots \\ \vdots & & \ddots & 0 \\ 0 & \cdots & & 1 \end{bmatrix}$$

In general, like the determinant, inverses take some work to calculate, and you should find a numerical routine.[6] For practice, however, it is useful to remember that the inverse of the 2×2 matrix

$$A = \begin{bmatrix} a & b \\ c & d \end{bmatrix}$$

is given by

$$A^{-1} = \frac{\begin{bmatrix} d & -b \\ -c & a \end{bmatrix}}{|A|}$$

Trace   The *trace* of a matrix A is the sum of its diagonal elements; that is,

$$Tr(A) = \sum_{i=1}^{N} a_{ii}$$

Positive Definite A matrix A is *positive definite* if for every x,

$$x^T A x > 0$$

and *positive semidefinite* if

$$x^T A x \geq 0$$

Orthonormal Transformation A transformation matrix A is orthonormal when

$$A^{-1} = A^T$$

As a consequence

$$A A^T = I$$

NOTES

1. A. P. Dempster, N. M. Laird, and D. B. Rubin, "Maximum Likelihood from Incomplete Data via the *EM* Algorithm," *Journal of the Royal Statistical Society, Series B* 39, no. 1 (1977): 1–22.

2. William H. Press et al., *Numerical Recipes in C: The Art of Scientific Computing*, 2nd ed. (New York: Cambridge University Press, 1992).

3. For a proof see David G. Luenberger, *Introduction to Dynamic Systems: Theory, Models, and Applications* (New York: Wiley, 1979).

4. Matthew Turk and Alex Pentland, "Eigenfaces for Recognition," *Journal of Cognitive Neuroscience* 3, no. 1 (1991):71–86.

5. Press, *Numerical Recipes in C*.

6. Ibid.

EXERCISES

1. For the vectors

$$x = \begin{pmatrix} 3 \\ 2 \\ 5 \end{pmatrix} \text{ and } y = \begin{pmatrix} -1 \\ 2 \\ -4 \end{pmatrix}$$

calculate
a. $\|x\|$
b. $x \cdot y$
c. The projection of x onto y

2. Show that

$$(AB)^{-1} = B^{-1} A^{-1}$$

3. A matrix is *orthonormal* if its columns v_i, $1 = 1, \ldots, n$ have the following property:

$$v_i \cdot v_i = 1$$

and for $i \neq j$

$v_i \cdot v_j = 0$

Show that for an orthonormal matrix A,

$A^T A = I$

4. For the matrix

$$\begin{bmatrix} 5 & -2 & 1 \\ 1 & 1 & 3 \\ 4 & -2 & 1 \end{bmatrix}$$

find (a) its trace and (b) its determinant.

5. Find the eigenvalues and eigenvectors of the matrix

$$\begin{bmatrix} -3 & 1 \\ 0 & -1 \end{bmatrix}$$

Could this matrix be the covariance matrix for some data? Say why or why not.

6. Find the eigenvalues and eigenvectors of the matrix

$$\begin{bmatrix} 4 & -1 \\ 2 & 1 \end{bmatrix}$$

Let Y be the eigenvector matrix and Λ the matrix

$$\begin{bmatrix} \lambda_1 & 0 \\ 0 & \lambda_2 \end{bmatrix}$$

for the vector

$$x = \begin{pmatrix} 3 \\ 4 \end{pmatrix}$$

a. What is y when $y = Wx$?
b. If $x^* = Y^{-1}x$ and $y^* = Y^{-1}y$, show that

$y^* = \Lambda x^*$

7. If v is an eigenvector of the matrix A and λ the associated eigenvalue, show that v is also an eigenvector of aA where a is a scalar. What is the corresponding eigenvalue?

8. Given the following two samples of some 5-dimensional data, find the two largest eigenvalues of the covariance matrix.

$$x = \begin{pmatrix} 3 \\ 2 \\ 7 \\ -1 \\ 4 \end{pmatrix} \text{ and } y = \begin{pmatrix} -1 \\ 2 \\ 2 \\ 6 \\ 3 \end{pmatrix}$$

9. Show that if a matrix A is symmetric and has distinct eigenvalues, its eigenvectors are orthogonal. Hint: If two vectors v_1 and v_2 are orthogonal, then from the eigenvector equation,

$$v_2^T A v_1 = \lambda_1 v_2^T v_1 = 0$$

10. Derive the version of the expectation-maximization algorithm when the data are in the form of vectors; that is,

$$x_i, i = 1, \ldots, n$$

11. Solve equations Equation 4.5 and 4.6 for expressions for m_k and σ_k in terms of the data points x_i.

5 Dynamics

ABSTRACT   All physical systems have inertia, and as a consequence the state vector is constrained to follow a smooth trajectory in state space. Motion in state space is known as the *dynamics* of the system. Such trajectories are best described differentially in terms of the rate of change of the state vector with time. The easiest systems to deal with are *linear systems*. These systems are completely characterized by their *eigenvalues* and *initial conditions*. Nonlinear systems can be approximated locally to stable equilibrium points, or *attractors*. In some cases their stability can be characterized by the behavior of trajectories with respect to values of a *Lyapunov function*.

5.1   OVERVIEW

Any physical system, such as neurons or muscles, will not respond instantaneously in time but will have a time-varying response termed the *dynamics*. The dynamics of neurons are an inevitable constraint of the times taken to charge cell bodies by ionic currents. Dynamics limit the ultimate speed of computation, but they also can be helpful. One way is to allow compact specifications for the generation of actions. Figure 5.1 shows an example of a trajectory used to write the letter A generated by the dynamics of a network of neurons.[1] If you were to generate this trajectory using a linear system such as described in Chapter 4, the only way to do it would be to describe every point on the trajectory. In contrast, a dynamical system allows just an initial point to be specified, and then it does the rest. For example, to generate the trajectory for the A, points on the letter are specified only during a training phase. After that, generating the trajectory shown in the figure requires only the starting point.

Dynamical systems can be described by several equations that can be summarized as a single vector equation

$$\dot{x} = F(x)$$

where $\dot{x}$, read as "x dot," denotes temporal derivative $\frac{dx}{dt}$ and, in vector notation,

$$x = \begin{pmatrix} x_1 \\ x_2 \\ \vdots \\ x_n \end{pmatrix} \text{ and } \dot{x} = \begin{pmatrix} \dot{x}_1 \\ \dot{x}_2 \\ \vdots \\ \dot{x}_n \end{pmatrix}$$

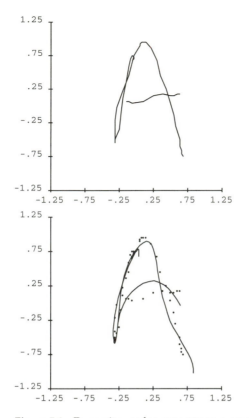

Figure 5.1 Dynamics used to generate an exemplar of the letter A. To generate this letter, a neural network is trained by being given examples of points along a trajectory, as shown in the upper part of the figure. The trajectory is actually a smooth curve conjoined with a "pen up/pen down" component of the state vector that signals when to write. The result of learning is that when given a static signal denoting the letter A, the natural time constants of the network's weights enable it to dynamically generate an exemplar. (From Simard, 1991.)

and

$$F(x) = \begin{bmatrix} f_1(x_1, x_2,..., x_n) \\ \vdots \\ f_n(x_1, x_2,..., x_n) \end{bmatrix} \tag{5.1}$$

where n is the *order* of the system. The dynamical system vector equation has a nice graphical interpretation. Where x is the position of the state vector, then $\dot{x}$ is its instantaneous velocity. And since $\dot{x} = F(x)$, then, for any point x, $F(x)$ describes the change in state of the system when started at x, as shown in Figure 5.2. By graphically following these arrows (equivalent to integrating the equation), the evolution of the system can be pictured.

Although the nonlinear system $\dot{x} = F(x)$ is difficult to solve in general, its behavior about *equilibrium points* can be very informative. Such points in the state space can be *stable*, wherein the state vector moves back after a

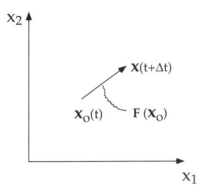

Figure 5.2 The dynamic function has a straightforward interpretation as the instantaneous direction of motion of the system in the state space.

perturbation, or *unstable*, wherein the state vector moves away after a perturbation.

Equilibrium point analysis can be formalized in terms of a linear approximation to the system at the point in question. The way to linearize a nonlinear system is to let $x = x_0 + \Delta x$ where x_0 is an equilibrium point. Then this equation can be expanded in a Taylor series (see appendix). Writing the terms up to first order explicitly and denoting the rest as higher-order terms (HOTs),

$$\dot{x}_0 + \Delta\dot{x} = F(x_0) + F'(x_0)\Delta x + \text{HOTs}$$

so that, since $\dot{x}_0 = F(x_0)$, and it is assumed that the HOTs can be neglected,

$$\Delta\dot{x} = F'(x_0)\Delta x \tag{5.2}$$

This system is linear, since the matrix $F'(x_0)$ is constant, being evaluated at the point x_0. This matrix $F'(x)$ is a matrix of *partial derivatives*, and is called the Jacobian, as shown in Eq 5.3:

$$F'(x) = \begin{bmatrix} \frac{\partial f_1}{\partial x_1} & \frac{\partial f_1}{\partial x_2} & \cdots & \frac{\partial f_1}{\partial x_n} \\ \frac{\partial f_2}{\partial x_1} & & & \\ \vdots & & & \\ \frac{\partial f_n}{\partial x_1} & \cdots & \cdots & \frac{\partial f_n}{\partial x_n} \end{bmatrix} \tag{5.3}$$

Example: Linearizing a Dynamical System For a second-order system let

$$F(x) = \begin{pmatrix} x_1 + x_2^2 \\ x_1 x_2 + x_2^2 \end{pmatrix}$$

Then the Jacobian is given by

$$F'(x) = \begin{bmatrix} 1 & 2x_2 \\ x_2 & x_1 + 2x_2 \end{bmatrix}$$

At equilibrium, $F(x) = 0$, so that the point $x_0 = \left(\begin{smallmatrix} -1 \\ 1 \end{smallmatrix}\right)$ is an equilibrium point. At this point the Jacobian $F'(x_0)$ simplifies to

$$F'(x_0) = \begin{bmatrix} 1 & 2 \\ 1 & 1 \end{bmatrix}$$

Equation 5.2 is crucial, since it turns out that the eigenvalues of the Jacobian matrix govern the dynamic behavior of the system. Where the approximation is exact, the eigenvalues describe the behavior for the entire state space. In the more general case of a nonlinear system, the approximation is local only to equilibrium points, but the eigenvalues are still extremely useful in predicting local behavior.

Models for Neuron Dynamics   A system of n neurons can be modeled by an equation of the form

$$\dot{x} = g(Wx)$$

where W is a matrix denoting synaptic connections and g is a function that prevents the value of x from becoming too large or too small. The linear form of the model is given by $\dot{x} = Wx$. Our ultimate objective is to describe ways of changing W to attain the dynamical behavior that achieves some goal, but before we can achieve it, we must understand how a given W governs dynamic behavior.

Another way of achieving dynamical trajectories is to "control" or "force" the system with a specific time-varying signal, perhaps generated by additional neurons. In this case the model of the system is extended to denote the *control* vector u:

$$\dot{x} = F(x, u)$$

As with the unforced case, insights into this system can be gained by studying its linear form,

$$\dot{x} = Ax + Bu$$

The distinction between achieving behaviors by changing W or changing u is that W is assumed to vary much more slowly than u whereas the latter is assumed to vary on a timescale with the state vector x.

5.2   LINEAR SYSTEMS

From the foregoing discussion you can appreciate that linear differential systems are important as an approximation to nonlinear systems. The reason for this importance is that they are easy to analyze. The solution to the general case can be obtained as the composition of the solutions to first- and second-order systems. Thus we start by solving these key examples.

Radioactive Decay The first example models the process of radioactive decay, as radioactive particles lose their radioactivity by emitting subatomic particles. The rate of this process is governed by the current amount of the substance.

Beginning with an amount M_0 of an element, and letting $x(t)$ denote the amount at any time t,

$$\dot{x} = -ax$$

To solve this expression, note that the equation is very close to setting the value of x equal to its derivative. This observation motivates trying e^t, since it is its own derivative. In fact, trying e^{ct},

$$ce^{ct} = -ae^{ct}$$

or

$$c = -a$$

so that e^{-at} is a solution.

Note that $x(t) = Ae^{-at}$ works for any A. This fact is fortunate because we have to be able to match the initial condition $x(0) = M_0$, since $e^0 = 1$, $A = M_0$, and $x = M_0 e^{-at}$.

Undamped Harmonic Oscillator The radioactive decay problem is an example of a first-order system as it can be described with a single scalar derivative. Figure 5.3 shows the classical second-order system of a spring and mass. Motion is constrained in the vertical direction. In the horizontal direction the only force is the spring force, which is a linear function of displacement, that is, $F = -kx$.

To derive the dynamic equation, start with Newton's law

$$F = ma$$

and substitute for the spring force. Acceleration is simply the second temporal derivative (in the notation "x double dot"):

$$-kx = m\ddot{x}$$

Rearranging,

$$\ddot{x} + \frac{k}{m}x = 0$$

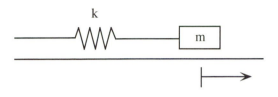

Figure 5.3 The classical second-order system: an undamped harmonic oscillator consisting of a mass connected to a spring. Of interest is the behavior of the system when the mass is displaced from the equilibrium point.

For the solution, as in the first-order case, try $x(t) = e^{at}$ so that

$$\ddot{x} = a^2 e^{at}$$

Substituting in the dynamic equation leads to

$$a^2 e^{at} + \frac{k}{m} e^{at} = 0$$

or, in other words,

$$a^2 = -\frac{k}{m}$$

Thus in this case the solution has imaginary roots; that is, where imaginary $i = \sqrt{-1}$,

$$a = \pm \sqrt{\frac{k}{m}} i$$

So the solution has the form

$$x(t) = Ae^{i\omega t} + Be^{-i\omega t}$$

where $\omega = \sqrt{\frac{k}{m}}$ and where A and B are constants that can be determined by the initial conditions. Assume the spring starts out with zero velocity and is stretched by d, then from the initial condition on position,

$$x(0) = d = Ae^0 + Be^0 = A + B$$

and next from the initial condition on velocity,

$$\dot{x}(0) = 0 = i\omega Ae^0 - i\omega Be^0$$

which implies that

$$A - B = 0$$

Combining these two equations in A and B,

$$A = B = \frac{d}{2}$$

Thus, finally, the solution is given by

$$x(t) = \frac{d}{2} e^{i\omega t} + \frac{d}{2} e^{-i\omega t}$$

This solution can also be written as a cosine. Recall Euler's formula,

$$e^{i\theta} = \cos\theta + i\sin\theta$$

which allows the cosine and sine to be expressed as

$$\cos\theta = \frac{e^{i\theta} + e^{-i\theta}}{2} \quad \text{and} \quad \sin\theta = \frac{e^{i\theta} - e^{-i\theta}}{2i}$$

so that $x(t) = d \cos \omega t$. What this result means is that you can forget about sine and cosine and consider only exponentials. An imaginary part of the exponential indicates an oscillation in the solution.

5.2.1 The General Case

Although the previous example is a second-order linear differential equation (LDE) with constant coefficients, it can be expressed equivalently as two first-order LDEs. To see this possibility, define

$$x_1 = x \quad \text{and} \quad x_2 = \dot{x}$$

Then

$$\begin{pmatrix} \dot{x}_1 \\ \dot{x}_2 \end{pmatrix} = \begin{bmatrix} 0 & 1 \\ -\dfrac{k}{m} & 0 \end{bmatrix} \begin{pmatrix} x_1 \\ x_2 \end{pmatrix}$$

The general form of this transformation, where $x_{n+1} = \frac{d^n x}{dt^n}$, works for LDEs with constant coefficients of *any* order. In other words, any nth-order LDE can be expressed as the sum of n first-order LDEs. The effect of this transformation is that the solutions that you studied for the first- and second-order case extend to the higher-order cases as well. For an n-dimensional vector, each component will either grow or decay exponentially, and it may oscillate as well if its exponent turns out to have an imaginary part. With this fact in mind, let us solve the general case, which is specified by

$$\dot{x} = Ax$$

where A is a matrix of constant coefficients.

How do we solve this system? Since $x = x_0 e^{at}$ worked before, try

$$x(t) = x_0 e^{At} \tag{5.4}$$

where x_0 is a vector of initial conditions. What about e^{At}? Since

$$e^x = 1 + x + \frac{x^2}{2!} + \frac{x^3}{3!} + \cdots$$

define e^A as

$$e^A \equiv I + A + \frac{A^2}{2} + \cdots$$

and substitute into both sides of $\dot{x} = Ax$:

$$Ax = A[I + At + \frac{(At)^2}{2!} + \frac{(At)^3}{3!} + \cdots]x_0$$

$$\dot{x} = [A + \frac{2A(At)}{2!} + \frac{3A(At)^2}{3!} + \cdots]x_0$$

Since these two are equal, as you can quickly verify, the solution defined by Eq 5.4 actually works. It's not practical to try and find it this way, as the series expansion of e^A is too cumbersome to work with, but suppose that the matrix A happened to be diagonal; that is,

$$A = \Lambda = \begin{bmatrix} \lambda_1 & & & 0 \\ & \lambda_2 & & \\ & & \ddots & \\ 0 & & & \lambda_n \end{bmatrix}$$

In this case, all the equations are decoupled and

$$e^A = e^\Lambda = \begin{bmatrix} e^{\lambda_1} & & & \\ & e^{\lambda_2} & & \\ & & \ddots & \\ & & & e^{\lambda_n} \end{bmatrix}$$

so that solving this system reduces to solving n versions of the one-dimensional case. That is,

$$x(t) = e^{At}x(0) = e^{\Lambda t}x(0) = \begin{bmatrix} x_1(0)e^{\lambda_1 t} \\ x_2(0)e^{\lambda_2 t} \\ \vdots \\ x_n(0)e^{\lambda_n t} \end{bmatrix}$$

Now remember from Chapter 4 that the matrix A can be diagonalized by a similarity transformation:

$$A^* = T^{-1}AT = \begin{bmatrix} \lambda_1 & & & 0 \\ & \lambda_2 & & \\ & & \ddots & \\ 0 & & & \lambda_n \end{bmatrix}$$

where T is the matrix of eigenvectors. This result motivates transforming x into a new coordinate system by

$$x^* = T^{-1}x$$

using

$$\dot{x} = Ax$$

Write

$$T^{-1}\dot{x} = T^{-1}ATT^{-1}x$$

that is,

$$\dot{x}^* = A^*x^*$$

Since A^* is diagonal, x^* has the simple solution format already described, that is,

$$\mathbf{x}^*(t) = \begin{bmatrix} x_1^*(0)e^{\lambda_1 t} \\ x_2^*(0)e^{\lambda_2 t} \\ \vdots \\ x_n^*(0)e^{\lambda_n t} \end{bmatrix}$$

To discover $x(t)$, use the fact that $x = Tx^*$.

This is the main conclusion: that the dynamics of an nth-order LDE with constant coefficients is completely characterized by its eigenvalues and eigenvectors. The eigenvector machinery developed in the previous chapter to find useful coordinates for groups of points in state space can be imported here and used to find the local motion of a particular point in state space.

Example Let the matrix A be given by

$$A = \begin{bmatrix} 1 & 2 \\ 1 & 3 \end{bmatrix}$$

Then

$$|A - \lambda I| = \lambda^2 - 4\lambda + 1 = 0$$

has the solution $\lambda = 2 \pm \sqrt{3}$. Thus T, which has the eigenvectors as columns, is given by

$$T = \begin{bmatrix} 1 & 1 \\ \dfrac{1 + \sqrt{3}}{2} & \dfrac{1 - \sqrt{3}}{2} \end{bmatrix}$$

and the solution is given by

$$\begin{pmatrix} x_1(t) \\ x_2(t) \end{pmatrix} = \begin{bmatrix} 1 & 1 \\ \dfrac{1 + \sqrt{3}}{2} & \dfrac{1 - \sqrt{3}}{2} \end{bmatrix} \begin{pmatrix} x_1^*(0)e^{(2+\sqrt{3})t} \\ x_2^*(0)e^{(2-\sqrt{3})t} \end{pmatrix}$$

Of course the initial conditions will be expressed in the original coordinate system and must be transformed into the * coordinate system by T^{-1}. This solution is summarized in Box 5.1.

5.2.2 Intuitive Meaning of Eigenvalues and Eigenvectors

Recall the graphical interpretation of $\dot{x} = F(x)$, shown in Figure 5.4. For a general nonlinear system there will be many equilibrium points, as implied by the diagram, but for a linear system $\dot{x} = Ax$ there is a single equilibrium point at the origin.

Box 5.1 Summary of the Solution of $\dot{x} = Ax$

Solve for the eigenvalues of

$$|\lambda I - A| = 0$$

Taking the determinant results in an nth-order characteristic equation in λ:

$$\lambda^n + a_1 \lambda^{n-1} + \cdots + a_{n-2} \lambda + a_{n-1} = 0$$

Solve this for $\lambda_1, \ldots, \lambda_n$. For each λ_i determine the eigenvector v_i from

$$[A - \lambda_i I]v_i = 0$$

At the end of the solution process, the answer is given by

$$x(t) = \sum_{i=1}^{n} a_i v_i e^{\lambda_i t}$$

where λ_i and v_i are the eigenvalues and eigenvectors of A and the a_i are determined by the initial conditions.

Notes:

1. Since the determinant $|A - \lambda_i I|$ is zero, the eigenvectors can be determined only up to a scale factor.

2. The solution method outlined here only works for distinct eigenvalues, that is, $\lambda_i \neq \lambda_j \; \forall i, j$. For multiple repeated roots, the solution method is more complex[2] and results in expressions of the form $t^n e^{\lambda t}$.

Let us study this point for a second-order system. Suppose that $\lambda_1 \neq \lambda_2$ and both λ_1 and λ_2 are real and negative. The v_1 and v_2 define directions along which a trajectory will move toward the origin, because along these lines $x = v$ and $\dot{v} = Av = \lambda v$. Away from these lines the trajectories will tend toward the origin, as shown in Figure 5.4a.[3]

Now suppose that $\lambda_1 \neq \lambda_2$ and both λ_1 and λ_2 are real and positive. The v_1 and v_2 define directions along which a trajectory will move away from the origin, again because along these lines $x = v$ and $\dot{v} = Av = \lambda v$. Away from these lines the trajectories will move outward but tend toward the eigenvector directions, as shown in Figure 5.4c.

Now suppose that λ_1 and λ_2 are complex conjugates. That is, $\lambda_1 = i\omega$ and $\lambda_2 = -i\omega$. In this case the state space trajectory will oscillate around the origin along an ellipse determined by the eigenvector directions, as shown in Figure 5.4b.

5.3 NONLINEAR SYSTEMS

Linear systems can be analyzed because the behavior over the entire state space can be determined. But nonlinear systems are more complicated, and their behavior can be analyzed only in the neighborhood of equilibrium points. Remember that these are the points for which

$$F(x) = 0$$

Linear systems are simple to characterize because they have a single equilibrium point. The behavior of a system is determined entirely by the values

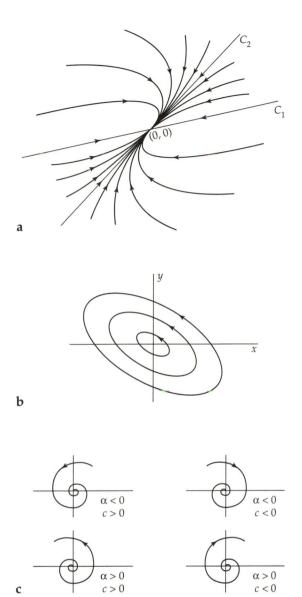

Figure 5.4 A nonlinear system may be understood by characterizing the behavior of trajectories of the system linearized near equilibrium points, as in this second-order system. This behavior is entirely determined by the eigenvalues and eigenvectors of the linearized system. (*a*) Two negative eigenvalues. (*b*) Two imaginary eigenvalues. (*c*) Complex eigenvalues whose real part, *a*, is negative or positive, as shown. (From Hurewicz, 1966 © MIT.)

of the eigenvalues and directions of the eigenvectors of the system. One of the main reasons that nonlinear systems, by far the general case, are not so easily handled is that they may contain multiple equilibrium points. How should they be analyzed?

The important realization is that characterizing the global behavior is too difficult and the best one can hope for is to characterize the behavior local to equilibrium points. The key issue is stability. One wants to know what will happen to the state vector when it is displaced from an equilibrium point. Broadly speaking, there are three kinds of behavior.

• Asymptotic stability: A displaced state vector will eventually return to the equilibrium point.

• Instability: A displaced state vector will continue to move away from the equilibrium point.

• Marginal stability: A displaced state vector will oscillate near the equilibrium point.

These concepts can be formalized as follows. First define a local region about the equilibrium point in terms of a sphere of radius R_0 centered at the point. The idea is that the analysis holds only for points inside this sphere because of nonlinear effects or other nearby equilibrium points.

An equilibrium point is *unstable* if for some R, $0 < R < R_0$, there is a sphere of smaller radius r that has the following property: There is a point inside $S(x, r)$ such that when started at that point, the state vector will eventually move outside of $S(x, R)$.

If an equilibrium point is not unstable, it is said to be stable, but that characterization does not mean a trajectory will tend toward the equilibrium point. For such a tendency to happen requires that the stronger condition of asymptotic stability be met. This condition is that in addition to being stable, there is some radius ρ such that when started inside $S(x, \rho)$, the trajectory will tend toward the equilibrium point.

An equilibrium point is marginally stable if it is stable but not asymptotically stable. Figure 5.5 shows these relations.

Stability analysis can proceed in two directions. One way is to resurrect the techniques for linear systems. If the location of an equilibrium point can be determined, then the dynamical equations can be linearized about that point and linear analysis applied. Another way is to find a special function of the state space, called a *Lyapunov function* (after its inventor). If the trajectory is such that the value of the Lyapunov function is always decreasing, then the dynamical system will be stable.

5.3.1 Linearizing a Nonlinear System

To see how the method of linearization can be used, consider the classic problem of the dynamics of animal populations. In particular, consider the case of two coexisting populations, one of deer and the other of wolves. The population of deer will grow unabated in the absence of a predator,

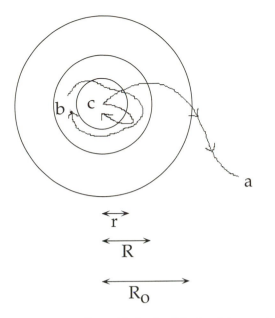

Figure 5.5   Different kinds of stability for state space trajectories: (*a*) unstable; (*b*) marginally stable; (*c*) asymptotically stable.

but will decline with the growth of the wolf population. Similarly, the population of wolves has a tendency to grow and needs the deer for food, so it will increase as a function of the deer population. These effects can be captured by the nonlinear differential equations[4]

$$\begin{pmatrix} \dot{x}_1 \\ \dot{x}_2 \end{pmatrix} = \begin{pmatrix} ax_1 - bx_1x_2 \\ -cx_2 + dx_1x_2 \end{pmatrix} \tag{5.5}$$

where a, b, c, and d are all assumed to be positive coefficients. For an equilibrium point, $\dot{x}_1 = \dot{x}_2 = 0$, so it is easy to see that this reasoning leads to an equilibrium point:

$$\begin{pmatrix} x_1 \\ x_2 \end{pmatrix} = \begin{pmatrix} \dfrac{c}{d} \\ \dfrac{a}{b} \end{pmatrix}$$

Now use Equation 5.2 to linearize Equation 5.5 about this equilibrium point. First compute the Jacobian,

$$F'(x) = \begin{bmatrix} a - bx_2 & -bx_1 \\ dx_2 & -c + dx_1 \end{bmatrix}$$

so the system at the equilibrium point is given by

$$\begin{pmatrix} \Delta \dot{x}_1 \\ \Delta \dot{x}_2 \end{pmatrix} = \begin{bmatrix} 0 & \frac{-bc}{d} \\ \frac{ad}{b} & 0 \end{bmatrix} \begin{pmatrix} \Delta x_1 \\ \Delta x_2 \end{pmatrix}$$

From this the characteristic equation is

$$\lambda^2 = -ac$$

so that the two roots are

$$\lambda_{1,2} = \pm\sqrt{ac}\, i$$

From the definitions of stability given earlier it is clear that this equilibrium point is marginally stable. When displaced from the equilibrium point, it will oscillate forever about that point without ever converging or becoming unstable. Thus a small increase in the deer population will result in a subsequent increase in the wolf population, which in turn will result in a subsequent decrease in the deer population, and so on.

5.3.2 Lyapunov Stability

The idea of Lyapunov stability is very beautiful. Suppose that you can pick a function that is in the shape of a bowl such that its lowest point is the equilibrium point. Call this function $V(x)$. If this function is decreasing in value as the trajectory progresses from all starting points near the equilibrium point, then the system is asymptotically stable. Why? If the trajectory continues to reduce the value of the chosen function, then eventually it must end up at the lowest point, which is the equilibrium point.

You can see that this function is like the ideas used to define stability at the beginning of this section. As Figure 5.6 shows, if the trajectory is always decreasing the value of $V(x)$, then the trajectory must always cross the level curves of V heading inward toward the equilibrium point. This relation is captured by the Lyapunov stability theorem (Box 5.2).

Formally this requirement is equivalent to the condition

$$\dot{V}(x) \le 0$$

To see this point, expand the derivative using the chain rule

$$\dot{V}(x) = \frac{\partial V}{\partial x_1}\dot{x}_1 + \frac{\partial V}{\partial x_2}\dot{x}_2 + \cdots + \frac{\partial V}{\partial x_n}\dot{x}_n$$

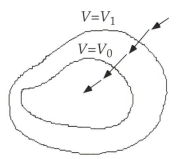

Figure 5.6 The idea behind Lyapunov stability. The state space trajectory always crosses level contours of V.

Box 5.2   Lyapunov Stability Theorem

> If there exists a Lyapunov function $V(x)$ for an equilibrium point x_o and region $X = S(x, R_0)$, then the equilibrium point is stable. Furthermore, if $\dot{V}(x) < 0$ for $x \neq x_o$, that is, if it is strictly negative everywhere except the equilibrium point itself, then the stability is asymptotic.

but remember that $\dot{x} = F(x)$, so that $\dot{V}(x)$ can be written as a dot product,

$$\dot{V}(x) = \nabla V \cdot F(x)$$

Formally, a function $V(x)$ is a Lyapunov function if over a region X of the state space that contains an equilibrium point x,

1. V is continuous and has continuous partial derivatives;
2. V has a single minimum at the equilibrium point;
3. $\nabla V \cdot F(x) \leq 0$ for all trajectories in X.

APPENDIX: TAYLOR SERIES

Vector notation provides a very compact way of expressing local approximations to functions. Recall that if a function and its derivatives are known at a particular point a, then it can be approximated near that point by the *Taylor series* formula. For a function of one variable this is

$$f(x) = f(a) + (x - a)f'(a) + \frac{(x - a)^2}{2!}f''(a) + \cdots$$

For vectors:

$$f(x) = f(x_0) + c^T(x - x_0) + \frac{1}{2}(x - x_0)^T A(x - x_0) + \cdots$$

where c is the vector

$$\left\{\frac{\partial f}{\partial x_i}\right\}_{x_0}$$

and A is the matrix

$$\left[\frac{\partial^2 f}{\partial x_i \partial x_j}\right]_{x_0}$$

The subscript x_0 means that the quantity in brackets is to be evaluated at $x = x_0$.

For example, if

$$f(x) = \begin{pmatrix} 2x_1^2 \\ x_2^3 + 3 \end{pmatrix} \quad \text{and} \quad x_0 = \begin{pmatrix} -3 \\ 2 \end{pmatrix}$$

then

$$c = \begin{pmatrix} 4x_1 \\ 3x_2^2 \end{pmatrix}_{x_0} = \begin{pmatrix} -12 \\ 12 \end{pmatrix}$$

and A is given by

$$A = \begin{bmatrix} 4 & 0 \\ 0 & 12 \end{bmatrix}$$

NOTES

1. This example is taken from Patrice Simard's Ph.D. thesis, "Learning State Space Dynamics in Recurrent Networks," TR 383, Computer Science Department, University of Rochester, 1991.

2. A book that explains this method is John C. Jaeger and Gordon Newstead's *An Introduction to the Laplace Transformation with Engineering Applications* (London: Methuen, 1969).

3. A discussion of the different cases is given in Witold Hurewicz's *Lectures on Ordinary Differential Equations* (Cambridge, MA: MIT Press, 1966).

4. The original formulation was due to Vito Volterra; for an English-language edition, see *Theory of Functionals and of Integral and Integro-Differential Equations* (New York: Dover, 1959).

EXERCISES

1. Much evidence has shown that the brain's motor system has internal oscillatory signals of about 10 cycles per second. Estimate how close piano playing and typing come to this limit by doing experiments.

2. If the speed of a hopping kangaroo is 30 kph and its stride is 10 meters, estimate its natural frequency.

3. For the dynamical system $\dot{x} = Ax$ where A is given by

$$\begin{bmatrix} 2 & 1 \\ 2 & 2 \end{bmatrix}$$

a. Solve this system given an initial condition

$$\begin{pmatrix} x_1(0) \\ x_2(0) \end{pmatrix} = \begin{pmatrix} 3 \\ 4 \end{pmatrix}$$

by transforming coordinates appropriately.

b. Make a *phase plot* of $[x_1(t), x_2(t)]$ starting from the initial condition.

4. Adding friction to the second-order spring-mass system results in the following dynamic equation:

$$m\ddot{x} + b\dot{x} + kx = 0$$

Transform this equation into a set of first-order equations and compute the eigenvalues of the system. For what values of b is the system stable?

5. The *Laplace transform* is useful because it allows the input/output relationship to be dealt with algebraically instead of in terms of differential equations and convolution integrals. The Laplace transform $F(s)$ of a scalar function of time $f(t)$ is defined by

$$\mathcal{L}[f(t)] = \int_0^\infty f(t)e^{-st}\,dt = F(s)$$

• $F(s)$ is a complex function of the complex variable s.

• The Laplace transform takes a function from the *time* domain (real) to the Laplacian domain (complex).

For example:

$$\mathcal{L}(e^{\lambda t}) = \int_0^\infty e^{\lambda t}e^{-st}\,dt$$

$$= \int_0^\infty e^{(\lambda-s)t}\,dt$$

$$= \left.\frac{e^{(\lambda-s)t}}{(\lambda - s)}\right|_0^\infty$$

$$= \frac{1}{s - \lambda}$$

[if $Re(\lambda) - Re(s) < 0$].
From the standpoint of dynamics, the most useful property of the Laplace transform is how it transforms the derivative.

$$\mathcal{L}\left(\frac{df}{dt}\right) = \int_0^\infty \frac{df}{dt}e^{-st}\,dt$$

since

$$\frac{d}{dt}(fe^{-st}) = \frac{df}{dt}e^{-st} - sfe^{-st}$$

so that

$$\int_0^\infty \frac{df}{dt}e^{-st} = \int_0^\infty \frac{d}{dt}(fe^{-st})\,dt + \int_0^\infty sfe^{-st}\,dt$$

$$= fe^{-st}\,|_0^\infty + s\int_0^\infty fe^{-st}\,dt$$

$$= -f(0) + sF(s)$$

This is especially useful as it is the basis for transforming differential equations to algebraic equations.

Assuming zero initial conditions, show that the standard set of linear differential equations $\dot{x} = Ax$ is equivalent to

$$[A - Is]X(s) = 0$$

6. Adding crowding to the basic predator-prey model results in an extra term that models the effect of the extra prey:

$$\dot{x}_1 = ax_1 - bx_1x_2 - ex_1^2$$

$$\dot{x}_2 = -cx_2 + dx_1x_2$$

a. Analyze the stability of this system. What is the type of the equilibrium point?

b. Assume that there are now two prey that compete for space. Formulate this model and linearize it. (You don't have to solve it!)

7. A second-order system has a dynamics described by

$$\dot{x} = F(x)$$

where

$$F(x) = \begin{bmatrix} -3x_1 + x_2^2 \\ -6x_1 + 12x_1x_2 \end{bmatrix}$$

a. What is its equilibrium point [other than (0, 0)]?

b. Is the equilibrium stable or unstable?

8. Use your knowledge of stability to suggest a model for epilepsy.

9. For a pendulum of subtended mass m and length l that is displaced by an angle θ, the dynamic equations are:

$$ml\ddot{\theta} + mb\dot{\theta} + mg \sin \theta = 0$$

Use $\omega = \dot{\theta}$ to transform this into a set of first-order systems and show that

$$V(\theta, \omega) = \frac{1}{2}ml^2\omega^2 + mgl(1 - \cos \theta)$$

is a Lyapunov function for this system.

10. For the dynamic system

$$\dot{x} = Ax$$

show that if A is symmetric and positive definite, then

$$V(x) = -x^TAx$$

is a Lyapunov function for the dynamic system. What does this imply about the eigenvalues of A?

6 Optimization

ABSTRACT Optimization theory is the engine of the learning algorithms that will appear in later chapters. All these algorithms work by searching a state space to make improvements in a function termed the *objective function*. A ubiquitous strategy, known as *gradient search*, is to follow the nearby rate of maximum improvement of the objective function. This rate can be computed by taking the derivative of the objective function with respect to the state space variables. While following the gradient, the system dynamic equations must be obeyed. The method of *Lagrange multipliers* allows the dynamic equations to be incorporated into the objective function.

6.1 INTRODUCTION

The central idea of natural computation is that the brain's programs can be thought of as "theories." These theories are valuable to the animal as they compress descriptions of the world, thereby increasing its behavioral repertoire. Our ultimate goal is to describe the learning algorithms that accomplish this purpose by working in an online mode. Here we take the final preparatory step.

Compressing data is equivalent to coming up with a shorter code for the data. Such a code can be discovered in many different ways, but the groundwork for choosing an objective function was laid in Chapter 2. Basically any function that reduces some measure of minimum description length is doing the right thing. Chapter 3 showed that an uninformed search of state spaces is prohibitively expensive. Optimization functions, or *objective functions*, in the form of entropy measures can make the search of such spaces practical by providing a "warmer or colder" function to guide paths through the state space.

The goal of this chapter is to describe the mechanics of minimizing an objective function. You might think that the essentials of this process were covered in Chapter 3, but several new elements have been introduced since then. The methods of Chapter 3 were predicated on states hardly ever being revisited. It's not that states could not be revisited. From the central position in the eight-puzzle problem, RIGHT, DOWN, LEFT, UP will get you right back where you started. And in chess, you can move pieces back to where they were before. In fact, repeating the same chess position three times constitutes a draw (tie). But repeated states were not utilized. Repeated states may strike you as an annoyance, but the notion of visiting the same state twice is central to learning. In order to do better, you have to realize what you did the last time, and, more importantly, that there was a last time! The fact that states repeat is actually a boon, as there are clever ways of exploiting this in the optimization process. The other new elements that have been introduced are the notion of a metric space wherein we can measure the distance between states, and the dynamics of the underlying system. These concepts serve to refine the notion of the state transition operator introduced in Chapter 3.

Combining the notion of repeated states with the constraint of the underlying dynamics leads to what is known as the *optimal control problem*. This is a very general problem of optimizing a functional that extends over time that is also subject to the constraints of a dynamical system.[1]

The optimal control problem can be described by introducing the system dynamics

$$\dot{x} = F(x, u)$$

which is assumed to start in an initial state given by

$$x(0) = x_0$$

and has controllable parameters u

$$u \in U$$

The objective function consists of a function of the final state $\psi[x(T)]$ and a cost function (or *loss function*) ℓ that is integrated over time.

$$J = \psi[x(T)] + \int_0^T \ell(u, x)\, dt$$

This concise statement of the problem will need a lot of unpacking to be properly understood, and the intent of this chapter is to do exactly that. We start by considering the simplest optimization problem, which is depicted in Figure 6.1:

$$\min_x \tilde{F}(x)$$

The next level of complication arises with the introduction of constraints. The simplest kind of constraint is an equality constraint, for example, $G(x) = 0$. Formally this addition is stated as

$$\min_x \tilde{F}(x) \text{ subject to } G(x) = 0$$

This complication can be handled by the *method of Lagrange*. This method reduces the constrained problem to a new, unconstrained minimization problem with additional variables. The additional variables are known as *Lagrange multipliers*. To handle this problem, add $G(x)$ to $\tilde{F}(x)$ using a Lagrange multiplier λ:

$$F(x, \lambda) = \tilde{F}(x) + \lambda G(x)$$

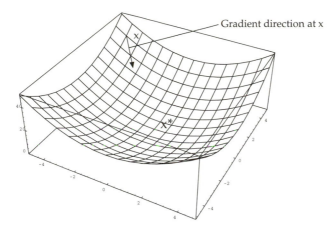

Figure 6.1 A simple case for optimization: a function of two variables has a single minimum at the point x^*.

Box 6.1 The Principle of Optimality

> From any point on an optimal state space trajectory, the remaining trajectory is optimal for the corresponding problem initiated at that point.

The Lagrange multiplier is an extra scalar variable, so the number of degrees of freedom of the problem has increased, but the advantage is that now simple, unconstrained minimization techniques can be applied to the composite function. The problem becomes

$$\min_{x, \lambda} F(x, \lambda)$$

Most often the equality constraint is the dynamic equations of the system itself, $\dot{x} = F(x, u)$, and the problem is to find an optimal trajectory $x(t)$. With this extension the problem assumes the generality of the optimal control problem. This problem may appear complicated at first glance, but there are two straightforward ways to solve it: (1) the method of Lagrange multipliers and (2) dynamic programming. We have already outlined the idea behind the Lagrange multipliers approach. The second way, dynamic programming, solves the constrained problem directly. The key is the *principle of optimality* (Box 6.1). This remarkably elegant observation leads to a simple way of solving the optimization problem directly that works especially well when all the variables are discrete.

6.2 MINIMIZATION ALGORITHMS

The techniques of this chapter are all directed toward finding a *local minimum*.[2] This can be done by starting from a point in the state space and making changes in the state vector that improve the objective function. There are two principal ways to do so.

One is to try for an algebraic solution. At the minimum $\frac{df}{dx} = 0$. We can calculate this derivative and attempt to solve for x. For example, if $f(x)$ is the following quadratic function

$$f(x) = 3x^2 + x - 4$$

taking the derivative

$$\frac{df}{dx} = 6x + 1 = 0$$

allows the direct solution of the extremum as

$$x = -\frac{1}{6}$$

This is a minimum because

$$\frac{d^2f}{dx^2} = 6 > 0$$

When $\mathbf{x}$ is a vector, the *Hessian* matrix A_n can be used to test for a maximum or minimum.[3] Where

$$A_n = \begin{bmatrix} f_{x_1^2} & f_{x_1 x_2} & f_{x_1 x_3} & \cdots \\ f_{x_2 x_1} & f_{x_2^2} & \cdots & \\ \vdots & & & \\ f_{x_n x_1} & \cdots & & f_{x_n^2} \end{bmatrix}$$

the condition for a minimum generalizes to a condition on the determinant of A_k, $k = 1, \ldots, n$, that is,

$$|A_k| > 0$$

for all $k = 1, \ldots, n$. Similarly, the condition for a maximum generalizes to

$$(-1)^k |A_k| < 0$$

for all $k = 1, \ldots, n$.

The second way of minimizing a function $f(x)$, which is of most practical importance in modeling biological systems, is to solve the problem iteratively using the gradient. Given a starting point and the derivative at that point, we can produce a new point that is closer to the desired minimum using

$$x^{new} = x^{old} - \eta \frac{df(x)}{dx}$$

The parameter η controls the size of the change in state vector and is very important. If it is too small, then the convergence to the optimum may be slow. If it is too large, then the algorithm may not converge at all.

Example: Minimizing a Quadratic   As an elementary example, let's re-consider the problem of finding the minimum of

$$f(x) = 3x^2 + x - 4$$

Pick a starting point of $x^{old} = 1$ and a learning rate of $\eta = 0.05$.

$$\frac{df}{dx} = 6x + 1$$

$$x^{new} = x^{old} - \eta\left(\frac{df}{dx}\right)_{x_{old}}$$
$$= 1 - 0.05(7) = 0.65$$

Repeating this calculation again shows that the estimate is approaching the minimum of $x = -0.16667$.

$$x^{new} = x^{old} - \eta\left(\frac{df}{dx}\right)_{x_{old}}$$
$$= 0.65 - 0.05(4.9) = 0.405$$

Example: A Single-Layered Network with Linear Activation   To start this modeling process, consider a single-layered network with two inputs and one output, as shown in Figure 6.2. The network uses the same linear summation activation function that was used in Chapter 4. Thus the output is determined by

$$y = \sum_k w_k x_k$$

The problem is to "train" the network to produce an output y for each of a series of input patterns x^p, $p = 1,\ldots, n$ such that the error between the desired output for each pattern, y^p, $p = 1,\ldots, n$ and the actual output y is minimized.

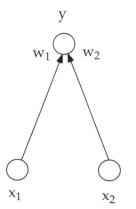

Figure 6.2   A simple case for optimization: a function of one variable minimizes error. Earlier a similar network was used to realize the computation of eigenvectors. There the weights for the network could be precomputed. Here they are determined by gradient descent.

The variables in this problem are the weights in the network. They are to be adjusted to minimize the error. Define an error function

$$E(w) = \frac{1}{2} \sum_p (y^p - y)^2$$

which is the same as

$$E(w) = \frac{1}{2} \sum_p \left(y^p - \sum_k w_k x_k^p \right)^2$$

One way to minimize the cost function $E(w)$ is to use gradient search. Starting from an initial guess use the derivative $\frac{\partial E(w)}{\partial w_k}$ to successively improve the guess.

$$w_k^{new} = w_k^{old} - \eta \frac{\partial E(w)}{\partial w_k}$$

The parameter η controls the size of the change at each step. The changes are discontinued when the improvements become very small. One way of measuring the improvement is $\sum_k \|w_k^{new} - w_k^{old}\| < \varepsilon$. For an appropriately chosen η this procedure will converge to a *local minimum* of $E(w)$.

Since E is a function of other variables besides w, the *partial derivative* is used in the preceding equation:

$$\frac{\partial E(w)}{\partial w_k} = -\sum_p (y^p - y) x_k$$

This is known as the *Widrow-Hoff learning rule*.

6.3   THE METHOD OF LAGRANGE MULTIPLIERS

Minimization is often complicated by the addition of constraints. The simplest kind of constraint is an equality constraint, for example, $G(x) = 0$. Formally this addition is stated as

$$\min_x \tilde{F}(x) \text{ subject to } G(x) = 0$$

The method of Lagrange reduces the constrained problem to a new, unconstrained minimization problem with additional variables. The additional variables are known as Lagrange multipliers. To handle this problem, append $G(x)$ to the function $\tilde{F}(x)$ using a Lagrange multiplier λ:

$$F(x, \lambda) = \tilde{F}(x) + \lambda G(x)$$

The Lagrange multiplier is an extra scalar variable, so the number of degrees of freedom of the problem has increased, but the plus side is that now simple, unconstrained minimization techniques can be applied to the composite function. The problem becomes

$$\min_{x, \lambda} F(x, \lambda)$$

Example: The Closest Point to a Circle   Find the closest point from the point (2, 2) to the circle $x^2 + y^2 = 1$. That is,

$$\min_{x,y} (x - 2)^2 + (y - 2)^2 \text{ subject to } x^2 + y^2 - 1 = 0$$

Solution.   Append the constraint using a Lagrange multiplier

$$\min_{x,\lambda} F(x, \lambda) = (x - 2)^2 + (y - 2)^2 + \lambda(x^2 + y^2 - 1)$$

Now differentiate with respect to variables x, y, and λ, and set the partial derivatives equal to zero for a local extremum.

$$F_x = 2(x - 2) + 2\lambda x = 0$$

$$F_y = 2(y - 2) + 2\lambda y = 0$$

$$F_\lambda = x^2 + y^2 - 1 = 0$$

Solve for x and y in the first two equations in terms of λ and substitute these solutions into the third,

$$\left(\frac{2}{1 + \lambda}\right)^2 + \left(\frac{2}{1 + \lambda}\right)^2 = 1$$

$$\lambda = 2\sqrt{2} - 1$$

So that finally,

$$(x, y) = \left(\frac{1}{\sqrt{2}}, \frac{1}{\sqrt{2}}\right)$$

Interpreting Lagrange Multipliers   Solving the unconstrained problem with the Lagrange multipliers is equivalent to solving the constrained problem. To see this, consider the problem

$$\min_{x,y} F(x, y) \text{ subject to } G(x, y) = 0$$

and suppose for a moment that the constraint equation could be solved so that

$$y = h(x)$$

In that case y can be eliminated from $F(x, y)$, reducing the problem to

$$\min_{x} F[x, h(x)]$$

which can be differentiated using the chain rule to obtain

$$F_x + F_y \frac{dy}{dx} = 0 \tag{6.1}$$

Now consider moving along the curve $G(x, y) = 0$. Let s be a parameter that varies with arc length so that $\frac{dG}{ds} = 0$, or alternatively

$$G_x \frac{dx}{ds} + G_y \frac{dy}{ds} = 0$$

Solving for $\frac{dy}{dx}$ and substituting into Equation 6.1,

$$F_x G_y = F_y G_x \tag{6.2}$$

So this equation must hold for the constrained problem. Now consider the unconstrained problem using the Lagrange multiplier,

$$F'(x, y, \lambda) = F(x, y) + \lambda G(x, y)$$

Differentiating with respect to x and y yields

$$F_x + \lambda G_x = 0$$

and

$$F_y + \lambda G_y = 0$$

Eliminating λ gives the desired result,

$$F_x G_y = F_y G_x$$

Thus the equation that defines the extrema in the unconstrained problem using Lagrange multipliers is the same as Equation 6.2, which was obtained by solving for the extrema in the constrained problem.

Equation 6.2 also has a nice interpretation in terms of geometry. Rewrite it as

$$\frac{F_x}{F_y} = \frac{G_x}{G_y}$$

What this says is that at the extremum, the gradient must be in the same direction as the gradient of level curves of $G = constant$. If this were not true, then one could improve F by sliding along $G = 0$ in the appropriate direction. This relationship is shown in Figure 6.3.

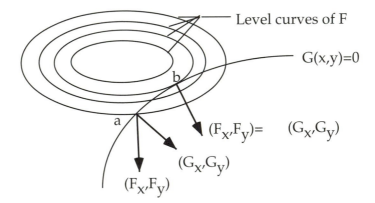

Figure 6.3 Interpretation of the constraint obtained by using Lagrange multipliers. At the local optimum point (b), $(F_x, F_y) = (G_x, G_y)$. At any other point, such as a, one can improve F by sliding along $G = 0$ in the appropriate direction.

6.4 OPTIMAL CONTROL

At last all the tools are in place to tackle the main problem of this chapter, the optimal control problem. Its beauty lies in its generality. All physical systems will have a dynamics with associated parameters. So a ubiquitous problem is to pick those parameters to maximize some objective function.

Formally the dynamics can be described by

$$\dot{x} = F(x, u)$$

which starts at an initial state given by

$$x(0) = x_0$$

and has controllable parameters u

$$u \in U$$

The objective function consists of a function of the final state $\psi[x(T)]$ and a function ℓ that is integrated over time.

$$J = \psi[x(T)] + \int_0^T \ell(u, x)\, dt$$

We will derive two principal ways of solving this problem that are at the core of the learning algorithms to come later. The first method is to extend the method of Lagrange multipliers. Things get a little tricky because of the integral in the formulation of J, but by being careful, we can derive differential equations that have to hold at the extrema, reminiscent of Section 6.3. This technique will be essential in Chapter 8. The second method works optimally for the case in which the state and control variables, x and u, are both discrete. This is the method of dynamic programming, a brute force method that directly solves these equations one step at a time. This technique will be essential for understanding the algorithms in Chapters 10 and 11.

6.4.1   The Euler-Lagrange Method

The goal of this section is to determine the conditions for the control to maximize the objective function J.

$$\max_u J \text{ subject to the constraint } \dot{x} = F(x, u)$$

The strategy will be to assume that u maximizes J and then use this assumption to derive other conditions for a maximum.[4] These arguments depend on making a perturbation in u and seeing what happens. Since u affects x, the calculations become a little involved, but the argument is just a matter of careful bookkeeping. The main trick is to add additional terms to J that sum to zero. Let's start by appending the dynamic equation to J as before, but this time using continuous Lagrange multipliers $\lambda(t)$:

$$\bar{J} = J - \int_0^T \lambda^T [\dot{x} - F(x, u)]\, dt$$

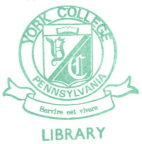

Anticipating what is about to happen, we define the *Hamiltonian* $H(\lambda, x, u)$ as

$$H(\lambda, x, u) \equiv \lambda^T [F(x, u)] + \ell(x, u)$$

so that the expression for $\bar{J}$ becomes

$$\bar{J} = \psi[x(T)] + \int_0^T [H(\lambda, x, u) - \lambda^T \dot{x}] \, dt$$

Now let's examine the effects of a small change in u on $\bar{J}$, as shown in Figure 6.4. Just keeping track of the change $\delta\bar{J} = J_v - J_u$,

$$\delta\bar{J} = \psi[x(T) + \delta x(T)] - \psi[x(T)]$$

$$+ \int_0^T [H(\lambda, x + \delta x, v) - H(\lambda, x, u) - \lambda^T \delta\dot{x}] \, dt$$

Using the expression for integration by parts[5] for $\int \lambda^T \delta\dot{x} \, dt$:

$$\int_0^T \lambda^T \delta\dot{x} \, dt = \lambda^T(T)\delta x(T) - \lambda^T(0)\delta x(0) - \int_0^T \dot{\lambda}^T \delta x \, dt$$

Now substitute this into the expression for $\delta\bar{J}$,

$$\delta\bar{J} = \psi[x(T) + \delta x(T)] - \psi[x(T)] - \lambda(T)^T \delta x(T)$$

$$+ \int_0^T [H(\lambda, x + \delta x, v) - H(\lambda, x, u) + \dot{\lambda}^T \delta x] \, dt$$

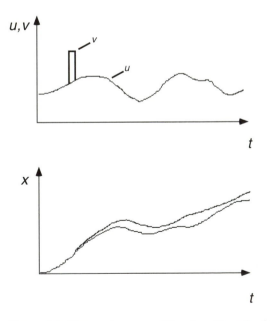

Figure 6.4 The maximum condition for $u(t)$ can be developed by studying a small perturbation about a trajectory that is assumed optimal. Where u results in x, v results in $x + \delta x$.

Now concentrate just on the first two terms in the integral:

$$\int_0^T [H(\lambda, x + \delta x, v) - H(\lambda, x, u)] \, dt$$

First add and subtract $H(\lambda, x, v)$:

$$= \int_0^T [H(\lambda, x + \delta x, v) - H(\lambda, x, v) + H(\lambda, x, v) - H(\lambda, x, u)] \, dt$$

Next expand the first term inside the integral in a Taylor series and neglect terms above first order,

$$\cong \int_0^T (H_x(\lambda, x, v)^T \delta x + H(\lambda, x, v) - H(\lambda, x, u)) \, dt$$

where H_x is the partial $\frac{\partial H}{\partial x}$, which is

$$\begin{pmatrix} H_{x_1} \\ \vdots \\ H_{x_n} \end{pmatrix}$$

Now add and subtract $H_x(\lambda, x, u)^T \delta x$:

$$= \int_0^T \left\{ H_x(\lambda, x, u)^T \delta x + [H_x(\lambda, x, v) - H_x(\lambda, x, u)]^T \delta x \right.$$
$$\left. + H(\lambda, x, v) - H(\lambda, x, u) \right\} dt$$

The term $[H_x(\lambda, x, v) - H_x(\lambda, x, u)]^T \delta x$ can be neglected because it is the product of two small terms, $[H_x(\lambda, x, v) - H_x(\lambda, x, u)]$ and δx, and thus is a second-order term. Thus

$$\cong \int_0^T \left(H_x(\lambda, x, u) \delta x + H(\lambda, x, v) - H(\lambda, x, u) \right) dt$$

Finally, substitute this expression back into the original equation for δJ, yielding

$$\delta \bar{J} \cong \left\{ \psi_x[x(T)] - \lambda^T(T) \right\} \delta x(T)$$

$$+ \int_0^T [H_x(\lambda, x, u) + \dot{\lambda}^T] \delta x \, dt$$

$$+ \int_0^T [H(\lambda, x, v) - H(\lambda, x, u)] \, dt$$

Since we have the freedom to pick λ, just to make matters simpler, pick it so that the first integral vanishes:

$$-\dot{\lambda}^T = H_x(\lambda, x, u)$$

$$\lambda^T(T) = \psi_x[x(T)]$$

So now all $\delta \bar{J}$ has left is

$$\delta \bar{J} = \int_0^T [H(\lambda, x, v) - H(\lambda, x, u)] \, dt$$

From this equation it follows that the optimal control u^* must be such that

$$H(\lambda, x, u^*) \geq H(\lambda, x, u), \, u \in U \tag{6.3}$$

To see this point, suppose that it were not true, that is, that for some interval of time there was a $v \in U$ such that

$$H(\lambda, x, v) \geq H(\lambda, x, u^*)$$

This assumption would mean that you could adjust the integral so that the perturbation $\delta \bar{J}$ is positive, contradicting the original assumption that $\bar{J}$ is maximized by u^*. Therefore Equation 6.3 must hold. This long but fruitful derivation has resulted in *conditions for optimality*, which are summarized in Box 6.2.

Example: Accelerating a Cart Consider the one-dimensional problem of accelerating a cart on a track, as shown in Figure 6.5. The problem is to pick a control law $u(t)$ that will get the cart as far as possible down the track at time T, but at the same time avoid costly accelerations.

The dynamic equation is

$$\ddot{x} = -\dot{x} + u(t)$$

with initial conditions

$$x(0) = 0$$

$$\dot{x}(0) = 0$$

Box 6.2 Summary of the Conditions for Optimality

In addition to the dynamic equations

$\dot{x} = f(x, u)$

and associated initial condition

$x(0) = x_0$

the Lagrange multipliers also must obey a constraint equation

$-\dot{\lambda}^T = H_x$

that has a *final condition*

$\lambda^T(T) = \psi_x[x(T)]$

The equation for λ is known as the *adjoint equation*. In addition, for all t, the optimal control u is such that

$H[\lambda(t), x(t), v] \leq H[\lambda(t), x(t), u(t)]$

where H is the Hamiltonian

$H = \lambda^T f(x, u) + \ell(x, u)$

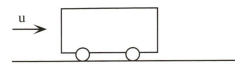

Figure 6.5 A cart on a one-dimensional track. The position on the track is given by $x(t)$. The cart is controlled by an acceleration $u(t)$.

The cost functional

$$J = x(T) - \frac{1}{2}\int_0^T u^2(t)\, dt$$

captures the desire to maximize the distance traveled in time T and at the same time penalizes excessive accelerations.

Using the transformation of Section 5.2.1, the state variables x_1 and x_2 are defined by

$$\begin{pmatrix} \dot{x}_1 \\ \dot{x}_2 \end{pmatrix} = \begin{pmatrix} x_2 \\ -x_2 + u \end{pmatrix}$$

$$x_1(0) = x_2(0) = 0$$

$$J = x_1(T) - \frac{1}{2}\int_0^T u^2\, dt$$

The Hamiltonian is given by

$$H = \lambda_1 x_2 - \lambda_2 x_2 + \lambda_2 u - \frac{1}{2}u^2$$

Differentiating this equation allows the determination of the adjoint system as

$$-\dot{\lambda}_1 = \frac{\partial H}{\partial x_1} = 0$$

$$-\dot{\lambda}_2 = \frac{\partial H}{\partial x_2} = \lambda_1 - \lambda_2$$

and its final condition can be determined from

$$\psi = x_1(T)$$

$$\lambda(T) = \psi_x(T) = \begin{pmatrix} 1 \\ 0 \end{pmatrix}$$

The simple form of the adjoint equations allows their direct solution. For λ_1,

$$\lambda_1 = \text{const} = 1$$

For λ_2, using the Laplace transform methods of Chapter 5,

$$\lambda_2 = 1 - e^{t-T}$$

For a maximum differentiate H with respect to u,

$$\frac{\partial H}{\partial u} = 0 \Rightarrow \lambda_2 - u = 0$$

$$u = \lambda_2 = 1 - e^{t-T}$$

So the optimal control is to start off with an acceleration of magnitude $1 - e^{-T}$ and then decrease it to 0 using the schedule presented here.

Linear System with Noise Up until now the state vector has been noise-less, but in any realistic case the state vector will be corrupted with noise. An especially elegant way of dealing with noise occurs when the system is linear. Suppose that the dynamic equation is given by

$$\dot{x} = Wx + \mu$$

where

$$x(0) = x_0$$

and where μ is a noise vector with parameters

$$E[\mu] = 0 \text{ and } E[\mu\mu^T] = Q$$

In other words, the state vector evolves from an initial condition and has noise added to it. The problem is to come up with an optimal estimate of the state that includes x and μ. How should we make this estimate? The state itself cannot be measured directly. Instead it is accessible through a measurement equation

$$z = x + v$$

where v is a noise vector with parameters

$$E[v] = 0 \text{ and } E[vv^T] = R$$

Thus one can only *estimate* the state. Lets call this estimate $\hat{x}(t)$. The covariance of the error in the estimate is then

$$P(t) = E\left[(x(t) - \hat{x}(t))^T(x - \hat{x}(t))\right]$$

and we will assume $P(0)$ is known.

Given an initial estimate $\hat{x}(0)$ we would like it to be close to the initial state, so $[\hat{x}(0) - x(0)]^T[\hat{x}(0) - x(0)]$ is a good measure. Similarly for the noise μ and measurements z we can use error metrics $\mu^T\mu$ and $(z - x)^T(z - x)$, respectively. The only additional wrinkle is to weight these measurements by the inverse of the covariance matrix. This step has the effect of making the term count less when its component is noisy. Thus the objective function is given by

$$J = \left[\hat{x}(0) - x(0)\right]^T P_0^{-1}\left[\hat{x}(0) - x(0)\right]$$

$$+ \int_0^T \left[\mu^T Q^{-1}\mu + (z - x)^T R^{-1}(z - x)\right] dt$$

The solution to this problem can be obtained from the optimality conditions. Where the Hamiltonian H is given by

$$H = \lambda^T(Wx + \mu) + \mu^T Q^{-1}\mu + (z - x)^T R^{-1}(z - x)$$

differentiating with respect to λ results in the dynamic equation

$$\dot{x} = Wx + \mu \tag{6.4}$$

Differentiating with respect to x results in

$$\dot{\lambda} = R^{-1}(z - x) - W^T \lambda \tag{6.5}$$

with final condition

$$\lambda(T) = 0$$

And finally, differentiating with respect to μ gives

$$\mu = Q\lambda \tag{6.6}$$

To solve this problem, postulate that the solution has the form

$$x = \hat{x} + P\lambda$$

with initial condition

$$x(0) = \hat{x}(0) + P(0)\lambda(0)$$

Differentiating this equation with respect to time and using Equations 6.4, 6.5, and 6.6 results in

$$-\dot{\hat{x}} + W\hat{x} + PR^{-1}(z - \hat{x}) = [-\dot{P} + WP + PW^T + Q - PR^{-1}P]\lambda$$

Since both sides of the equation are independent, they must be independently zero, that is,

$$\dot{\hat{x}} = W\hat{x} + PR^{-1}(z - \hat{x}) \text{ with } \hat{x}(0) = \hat{x}_0 \tag{6.7}$$

and

$$\dot{P} = WP + PW^T + Q - PR^{-1}P \text{ with } P(0) = P_0 \tag{6.8}$$

Equation 6.8 is known as the Ricatti equation.

Thus the optimal estimate of the state can be obtained by first solving the Ricatti equation to get $P(t)$ and then using it to solve Equation 6.7.

6.4.2 Dynamic Programming

The second main method of solving the optimal control problem is a direct method that works best for discrete systems. The first step is to convert the formulation of the problem to a discrete $x(k)$ and $u(k)$, $k = 0,..., N - 1$.

The dynamics are now expressed by a difference equation,

$$x(k + 1) = f[x(k), u(k)]$$

The initial condition is:

$$x(0) = x_0$$

The allowable control is also discrete:

$$u(k) \in U, k = 0,..., N$$

Finally, the integral in the objective function is replaced by a sum:

$$J = \psi[x(T)] + \sum_{0}^{N-1} \ell[u(k), x(k)]$$

To solve this equation directly, recall that the principle of optimality states that from any point on an optimal trajectory, the remaining trajectory is optimal for the corresponding problem initiated at that point. A way of using this principle is to start at one time step just before the end, that is, at $k = N - 1$, and calculate the best control for each possible state $x(k)$. Once this calculation has been done, back up one step to $k = N - 2$. The principle states that the steps from $k = N - 1$ should be part of the solution so that they can be utilized in building the optimal solution from step $N - 2$. Along the way, partial results of what is the best thing to do must be kept for every point in the state space that is examined. Let us let $V(x, k)$ keep track of these partial results.

Now it's easy to see that at the end,

$$V(x, N) = \psi[x(N)]$$

One step back,

$$V(x, N - 1) = \max_{u \in U} \left\{ \ell[u(N - 1), x(N - 1)] + \psi[x(N)] \right\}$$

And in general, for $k < N - 1$,

$$V(x, k - 1) = \max_{u \in U} \left\{ \ell[u(k - 1), x(k - 1)] + V[x(k), k] \right\}, k = 0,..., N$$

These equations are elegant in their simplicity but suffer from the "curse of dimensionality," in that as the state space increases in size, the amount of memory needed for V increases as M^d, where M is the discretization used for each state variable and d is the dimension of the space. The extent of the calculations can be appreciated by consulting Figure 6.6. The first pass in dynamic programming is the calculation of the objective function or value $V(x, k)$ for each point in the state space and for each discrete time, from $k = 1,..., T$. The top part of this figure shows the calculations proceeding backward in time. From the penultimate state you can try out all the possible controls and pick the one that best maximizes $V[x(k - 1), k - 1]$. Next the calculations are repeated for the state space at $k - 2$ and so on, back to the initial time $k = 0$. Along the way the values of u that maximize V are saved. Next, at time $k = 0$, the recovery of the best control starts with the recovery of the best control for the particular initial condition $x(0)$. That u generates the state $x(1)$, and the best control from that state is recovered. The recovery of the trajectory proceeds until the final time is reached, as shown in the lower part of the figure.

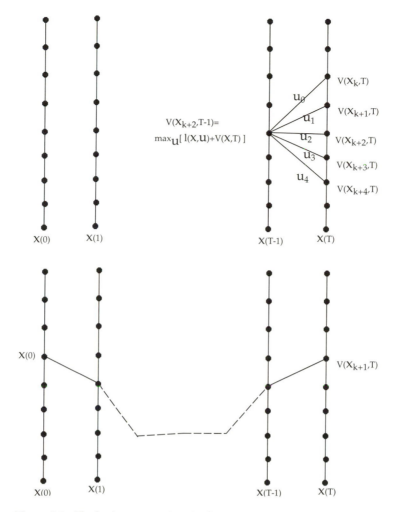

Figure 6.6 The basic computations in dynamic programming can be seen as a stage-wise process that starts at the terminal time and proceeds back to the initial time. (*upper*) The computation of the value for each node in the state space. During this calculation the control that produces the best value is also saved. (*lower*) At the end of the calculation, the remembered best controls can be used to recover the state space trajectory.

Example: The Cart Revisited   Consider a simple version of the cart problem where the state equations are given by

$$x(k + 1) = x(k) + v(k)$$

$$v(k + 1) = v(k) + u(k)$$

and the cost function is

$$J = x(T) - \sum_{0}^{N-1} \frac{u(k)^2}{2}$$

with $T = 9$ and $N = 9$.

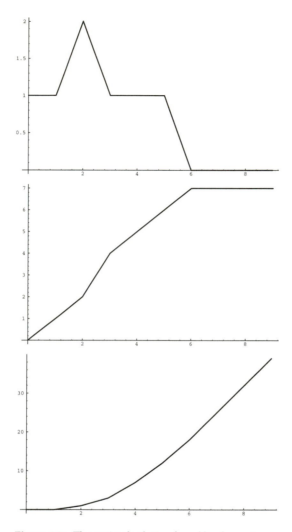

Figure 6.7 The optimal solution found by dynamic programming: (*top*) acceleration profile; (*middle*) velocity profile; (*bottom*) distance profile.

The results are shown in Figure 6.7a–c. Note that the different form of the dynamic equations results in a solution that is slightly different from the one found analytically using the Hamiltonian. However, the qualitative features of the solution are the same: Accelerate the cart at the beginning and then back off at the end.

NOTES

1. The phrase "optimal control problem" dates from the 1960s, when this corpus of mathematics was refined for use in rocket launch guidance systems. But the basic mathematics was developed much earlier by Euler and Lagrange. Frederick Y. M. Wan, *Introduction to the Calculus of Variations and Its Applications* (New York: Chapman and Hall, 1995); Enid R. Pinch, *Optimal Control and the Calculus of Variations* (New York: Oxford University Press, 1993).

2. The function $f(x)$ has a *local minimum* at the point x^* if $f(x^*) \le f(x)$ if $\|x^* - x\| < \varepsilon$ where the distance metric is Euclidean distance defined earlier, that is, $\|x\| = (\sum x_i^2)^{1/2}$.

For a local minimum we have the intuition that the function looks somewhat like a bowl. This is captured formally by first constraining the local domain of the function and then constraining the range of the function.

- A region R is *convex* if and only if

$x_1 \in R$ and $x_2 \in R \Rightarrow$

$x = \lambda x_1 + (1 - \lambda)x_2 \in R$ for all λ s.t. $0 < \lambda < 1$

- A function $f(x)$ is convex if and only if

when $x = \lambda x_1 + (1 - \lambda)x_2$, then

$f(x) \le \lambda f(x_1) + (1 - \lambda)f(x_2)$

- If R is convex and $f(x)$ is convex on R, then any local minimum is also a global minimum.

3. The Hessian can also be related to convexity. The function $f(x)$ being convex is equivalent to $x^T A x \ge 0$ for all $x \ne 0$.

4. This development essentially follows that of David G. Luenberger, *Introduction to Dynamic Systems: Theory, Models, and Applications* (New York: Wiley, 1979).

5. Recall that $d(uv) = u\,dv + v\,du$, so it follows that $uv = \int u\,dv + \int v\,du$.

EXERCISES

1. Find the point on the line $x + y = 1$ that maximizes the function $f(x, y) = 2x^2 + 3y^2$ using the method of Lagrange multipliers.

2. For the function

$$f(x_1, x_2) = x_1^2 - x_1 x_2 + 3x_2^2$$

find the minimum using the gradient method. Show all steps.

3. Given a cube of edge a, the problem is to drill a cylindrical hole of depth h and radius r such that the surface area of the hole is $5/16\pi a^2$, and the volume of the remaining solid is minimized (see Figure 6.8).

a. Use the method of Lagrange multipliers to solve this problem.

b. Use the constraint to reduce the problem to minimize a function of one variable.

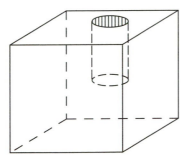

Figure 6.8 A cube with a cylindrical hole.

4. The brain registers an image I of n samples total. Suppose that in the brain there are m neurons represented by a vector r whose job it is to predict the intensity values of an image. The way they make this prediction is by acting through $n \times m$ synaptic weights W such that the predicted image is given by

$$I' = Wr$$

Furthermore the cost of representing this reconstruction is given by

$$a\|r\|^2 + \beta\|W\|^2$$

where a and β are constants and $\|\cdot\|^2$ means the sum of the squares of the individual elements regardless of whether they comprise a vector or matrix.

Given that you want to minimize both reconstruction error $\|I - I'\|^2$ and cost, derive the formula that will change the values of the individual elements of W according to a gradient descent rule.

5. Find the best dimensions (radius and height) for a can of constant surface area A. Check that your value is a maximum by using the Hessian.

6. Use the method of Lagrange multipliers to show that the probabilities that maximize the entropy

$$H = -\sum_{i+1}^{n} p_i \log p_i$$

are all equal, and that the resultant value of H is $\log n$.

7. Recall from Section 4.4.2 that

$$d^2(\mathbf{Z}, 0, \Sigma) = \mathbf{Z}^T \Sigma^{-1} \mathbf{Z}$$

Use the method of Lagrange multipliers to find a $\mathbf{Z}$ such that $\mathbf{Z}^T\mathbf{Z} = 1$ and $d^2(\mathbf{Z}, 0, \Sigma)$ is maximized. Show that

$$\Sigma\mathbf{Z} = \lambda\mathbf{Z}$$

in other words, that the optimal $\mathbf{Z}$ is an eigenvector of the covariance matrix.

8. Derive the optimal estimate $\hat{x}$ for the case where

$$\dot{x} = w$$

$$z = x + v$$

$$P(0) = p, \quad Q = q, \quad R = r$$

$$\hat{x}_0 = a$$

9. Suppose the dynamic equation for the cart is now $\ddot{x} = u$. How does this change the answer? Show all steps.

10. Consider the problem of optimizing a linear system with quadratic costs. That is, the system equation is given by

$$\dot{x} = Wx + u$$

with initial condition

$$x(0) = x_o$$

and costs are measured by

$$J = \psi\left[x(T)\right] + \int_0^T \left[x^T A x + u^T B u\right] dt$$

a. Use the method of solution for the Kalman filter problem to solve this problem also.

b. Comment on the significance of the relationship between the Kalman filter problem and this problem.

II   Memories

A basic and crucial function of the brain is to compute appropriate responses to complex situations quickly. In deciding to run from tigers there is not much time. How quickly can this decision be made? Chapter 1 showed that the fastest time for deciding is about 50 milliseconds. This result can be obtained from two sources. The first is an argument from the principles of the underlying circuitry. Alan Newell argued that the circuitry that has to support such a computation has to take about 10 ms, and there will also be the overhead of implementing the more complex computation. The 50-ms figure can also be observed from numerous psychological experiments, which show that if less than this time is allocated to displaying a visual input,[1] the human subject will not be able to recognize it. Also, searching an array of visual tokens takes about 50 ms per token.[2]

In 50 ms there is little else to do but have the right response pre-stored and look it up. Hence, at this timescale, the brain, most noticeably the cortex, is seen as a huge memory, or look-up table. Look-up tables can be seen as a way of storing correct reactions to situations. A stimulus pattern is sensed, and a response must be generated immediately.

THE CORTEX AS A HIERARCHICAL MEMORY

In broad terms the cortex is organized hierarchically, as shown in Figure II.1. The sensory input is transformed in a series of stages into invari-

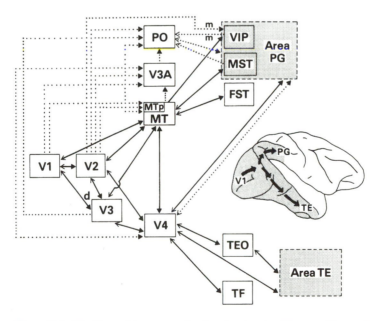

Figure II.1 The hierarchies composing the visual cortex. The overall organization of the cortex is hierarchical, as exemplified by the visual system. The incoming signal is split into two broad functional categories and processed in a stage-wise manner to compute increasingly abstract invariants. (From Robert Desmione and Leslie G. Underleider, "Neural Mechanisms of Visual Processing in Monkeys," in F. Boller and J. Grafman, eds., *Handbook of Neuropsychology*, vol. 2 [Amsterdam: Elsevier Science, 1989, pp. 267–99].)

Table II.1 The function of different cortical areas.

Location Pathway		Identification Pathway	
Area	Function	Area	Function
FEF	Target position	IT	Target identity: faces
MST	Target tracking	V4	Feature invariants
MT	Motion processing	V2	Surfaces
V2	Surfaces	V1	Photometric stimulus
V1	Photometric stimulus		

ants. These are then elaborated into motor commands by a reverse process. The most is known about the visual cortex, which probably can serve as a model for the other cortices. The visual cortex begins with area V1, which contains a retinotopic map of the visual field. Each hemisphere represents approximately a hemifield. This retinotopic map is connected to a similar map termed V2. Subsequent connections to other maps are organized hierarchically,[3] as shown in the figure.

In concert with the anatomical evidence is evidence from numerous other sources, such as neurophysiological recordings from animals and functional imaging of humans. This reinforces the central idea that the cortex represents information hierarchically. This evidence is summarized in Table II.1.

With respect to our 50-ms timescale, what are the computational problems that the memory has to solve in order to function? There are two broad classes of problems that must be solved.

• **Computing Invariants**.   This is a complex coding problem. One wants to associate all the different ways a tiger appears in an image with the internal state "tiger."

• **Completing Partial Patterns**.   As part of this problem the input information may be incomplete or mathematically underdetermined. There must be some way of correcting the encoding for "errors."

NEURAL NETWORK MODELS

To make progress, you need to settle on a model of a neuron that neglects some features and emphasizes others that you think are important. The standard model is shown in Figure II.2. To avoid confusing a biological neuron's many other features with the model neuron, we'll call the model neuron a *unit*.

The *state* of a unit models the firing rate. This is captured by a real number that ranges between 0 (inhibited) and 1 (firing furiously, say at 100–500 spikes per second). The weight w_{ij} between unit j and unit i will be a signed real number that models the effects of a synapse. Let us restrict our attention to digital units.

The way of changing the state vector specifies a *dynamics* for the system. The equation one might first think of using is

$$x_i = \sum_j w_{ij} x_j \qquad\qquad (II.1)$$

The problem with this is that x_i could be arbitrarily large. To restrict it to lie between 0 and 1, let us use a limiting function:

$$\sigma(x) = \frac{1}{1 + e^{-x}}$$

This function is shown in Figure II.3.

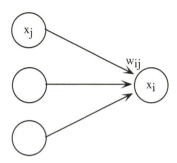

Figure II.2 The basic neural network model consists of neurons that represent a state. Units are connected via weights.

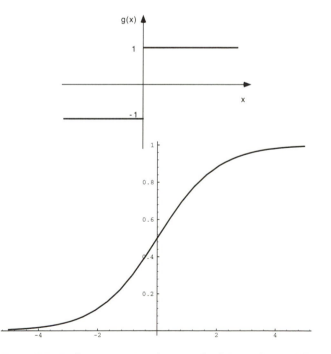

Figure II.3 Different activation functions lend themselves to different kinds of models. The threshold function is most easy to analyze, whereas the sigma function, being differentiable, lends itself to the propagation of subtle differences.

Thus Equation II.1 becomes

$$x_i = \sigma\left(\sum_j w_{ij} x_j\right)$$

A large number of interconnected units is a *network*. If a large number of units are interconnected in a network, one can describe the state of the network in terms of a state vector x. This just has the states of individual units as components, that is, for n units, $x = (x_1, x_2, x_3, \ldots, x_n)$.

Networks can be connected together in different ways, or different *topologies*. This fact turns out to be crucial in mathematical modeling, as different mathematical models are possible with different networks. For the problem of filling in gaps, networks with symmetric connections have proved the most useful. For the problem of computing invariants, feedforward networks, such as that shown in Figure II.4, have proved the most useful.

The ultimate goal is to specify the weights so that the changes in the state vector can be used as an algorithm to solve problems.

Content-Addressable Memory

Content-addressable memory (CAM) is a way of learning the patterns such that the patterns can be highly noise tolerant. In other words, they can be distorted and have missing parts. The job of a CAM is to fill in the missing parts appropriately (Figure II.5). That is, the input pattern is corrected to the nearest remembered pattern using some distance measure.

Supervised Learning

A way of creating such patterns is through learning from examples. The examples may come with a *label*, indicating the correct response, or the data may be *unlabeled*. The two cases are called supervised and unsupervised, respectively. The basic CAMs do not exhibit any generalization.

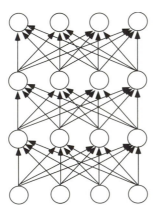

Figure II.4   A layered feedforward network contains no cycles.

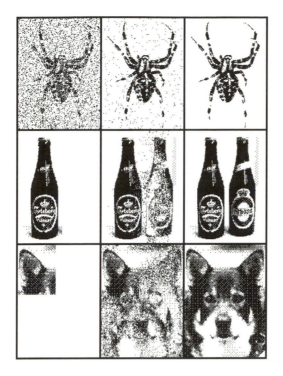

Figure II.5 Content-addressable memory fills in missing details. (From John Hertz, Anders Krogh, and Richard G. Palmer, *Introduction to the Theory of Neural Computation*, Volume 1 [figure 2.1 from p. 12], © 1991 Addison-Wesley Publishing Company, Inc. Reprinted by permission of Addison-Wesley Longman, Inc.)

Generalization allows the system to recognize similar patterns as instances of the same situation. Supervised methods are ways of clustering the data according to their projected use in addition to their intrinsic organization. The best of these methods uses an error function between the classification produced by the network and the desired classification to improve the classification incrementally.

Unsupervised Learning

Supervised learning is an attractive model only in restricted circumstances. For most biological systems, realistic learning models must be predominantly data driven. The prototypes formed are functions of the data distribution of patterns. We focus on one of the best unsupervised methods, Kohonen learning. Kohonen learning represents instances of patterns efficiently with stored prototypes.

NOTES

1. For example, see M. I. Posner and S. E. Petersen, "The Attention System of the Human Brain," *Annual Review of Neuroscience* 13 (1990):25–42.

2. A. Treisman, "Features and Objects," 14th Bartlett Memorial Lecture, *Quarterly Journal of Experimental Psychology* 41A (1988):201–37.

3. The hierarchical connections were determined anatomically by many researchers, notably Van Essen and Allman: D. Van Essen and J. H. R. Maunsell, "Hierarchical Organization and Functional Streams in the Visual Cortex," *Trends in Neurosciences* 6 (1983):370–75; J. Allman, "The Origin of the Neocortex," *Seminars in the Neurosciences* 2 (1990):257–62. The cortex as a whole is a two-dimensional sheet of cells arranged in distinct layers. The top layers are for processing; the middle layers are for input, from other cortical areas or other parts of the brain; and the bottom layer is for output, to other parts of the cortex or to the brainstem. If an area A is more abstract than an area B, its output neurons will connect to the upper and lower layers of B. In contrast, B's connections to A will terminate in A's input layer. Thus by comparing the gross features of connections between areas, a hierarchy can be established.

7 Content-Addressable Memory

ABSTRACT   Conventional silicon memory has a separate address and contents. This characteristic facilitates the reuse of the memory but makes it expensive to find a given item. In contrast, biological memory models abandon reusability in favor of fast accessing strategies. These strategies use the contents of the memory to also play the role of the address, hence *content-addressable memories.* The two principal types of such memories are *Hopfield memories* and *Kanerva memories.* Content-addressable memories are usually autoassociative—they fill in a partially specified memory—but they can also be heteroassociative—associating one pattern with another. Hopfield memories are autoassociative, but Kanerva memories can be both autoassociative and heteroassociative.

7.1   INTRODUCTION

Think of looking up a number in the phone book. The telephone book is organized by surname, so the first step is to know the surname of the person whose number you need. Here the surname plays the special role of the address or, in database parlance, the *key.* In the same way conventional silicon memory is distinguished by having separate addresses and contents. Thus the assignment $x := 3$ is understood as replacing the contents of the location specified by x with the value 3. This separation is very different from one way that we think the brain works, which is by using the contents as the address itself. The crucial idea is that any part of the information of the desired record can be used as a key. A *content-addressable memory (CAM)* will fill in the rest to recover the complete record.

You already covered the basic ideas behind the workings of a CAM when you studied nonlinear dynamics. A linear system has a single equilibrium point at the origin, but a nonlinear system may have many such points. A CAM is a nonlinear system with many such points that are all (or almost all) stable. Thus, when the state space vector is near such a point, it will be drawn to that point by the dynamics of the system. For that reason stable equilibrium points are called *attractors.* The amount of specificity in the initial condition of the state vector, the key, determines how close that point is to its attractor initially.

We will study two kinds of CAM. The first kind is *Hopfield memories.* These have an attractively simple structure in that the procedures for setting them up require little more than the patterns to be stored. They can solve tasks such as the phone book example. Hopfield memories are autoassociative;

they can recover the pattern stored given a portion of the pattern as input. What they cannot do is provide heteroassociative memories in which one pattern is recovered as a function of another. For that, we will need the additional machinery of *Kanerva memories*. Kanerva memories are heteroassociative, and have a number of other attractive properties as well. In addition, they can be seen as a generalization of Hopfield memories.

While the construction of silicon memory is very well understood, the exact structure that provides biological memory is very poorly understood. Nonetheless, to make progress, we have to start somewhere. The hypothesis that will guide us is that an abstraction of a neuron will represent a memory bit.[1] This abstraction needs some additional structure to set the value of the bit. The model of a neuron that is widely used for this purpose is shown in Figure 7.1. The model neuron is much simpler than a real neuron, so to avoid confusing a biological neuron's many other features with the model, we'll call the model neuron a *unit*. A large number of interconnected units is a *network*. The *state* of a unit will be discrete, either 1 or -1. (In later chapters an analog state of a real number between 0 and 1 will be very important, but here the ± 1 state is the easiest to work with; it will simplify the analysis.)[2]

The key parameters that define the memories are the weights. These model synaptic connections between units, as shown in Figure 7.1. Biological synapses are very complicated, so modeling them with a single real number is a gross simplification. The goal is to specify the weights so that the changes in the state vector can function as a memory. The weight w_{ij} between unit j and unit i will be a signed real number.

If a large number of units are interconnected in a network, one can describe the state of the network in terms of a state vector x. This just has the states of individual units as components; that is, for N units, $x = (x_1, x_2, x_3, \ldots, x_N)$.

The next step is to define a way of changing the state vector. This specifies a dynamics for the system. The equation one might first think of using is to make the state linearly dependent on the product of the input and synaptic weights:

$$x_i(t + 1) = \sum_{j=1}^{N} w_{ij} x_j(t) \qquad (7.1)$$

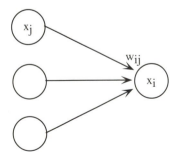

Figure 7.1 The fundamental abstraction of a neuron represents the state of each neuron i as a firing rate x_i and the synapse connecting neurons i and j as a real numbered weight w_{ij}.

Chapter 7   Content-Addressable Memory

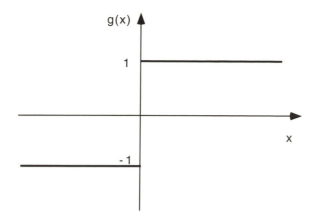

Figure 7.2 A standard activation function for neural units.

The problem with this equation is that x_i could be arbitrarily large. To restrict it to be either ± 1, let us use a limiting function:

$$g(x) = \begin{cases} +1 & x \geq 0 \\ -1 & \text{otherwise} \end{cases}$$

This function is simply the sign of its argument and is shown in Figure 7.2. Thus Equation 7.1 becomes

$$x_i(t + 1) = g\left(\sum_{j=1}^{N} w_{ij} x_j(t)\right)$$

7.2 HOPFIELD MEMORIES

Hopfield memories are networks in which every unit is connected to all the others. Furthermore, the weights connecting the units are symmetric; that is, $w_{ij} = w_{ji}$. It turns out that, for any given problem, it is relatively easy to pick w_{ij} so that the network will act like a memory. Given a set of Q patterns to be stored x^p, $p = 1, \ldots, Q$, the appropriate setting for the weights is given by

$$w_{ij} = \sum_{p=1}^{Q} x_i^p x_j^p \tag{7.2}$$

This is a form of a Hebbian Rule,[3] which makes the weight strength proportional to the product of the firing rates of the two interconnected units. You might also recognize this as the correlation matrix of the patterns. Writing the weights as a matrix makes this obvious:

$$W = \sum_{p=1}^{Q} x^p (x^p)^T$$

Example As an example of the weight calculation, pick the following three patterns to be stored in a memory:

In this case $Q = 3$ and let

$$x^1 = (-1, 1, 1, -1, \ldots)^T$$
$$x^2 = (1, 1, -1, -1, \ldots)^T$$
$$x^3 = (-1, 1, -1, 1, \ldots)^T$$

Now calculate one of the weights, for example, w_{23}:

$$w_{23} = x_2^1 x_3^1 + x_2^2 x_3^2 + x_2^3 x_3^3$$
$$= (1 \times 1) + (1 \times -1) + (1 \times -1) = -1$$

Note that the formula for the weights allows the weights to be adjusted incrementally with each new pattern; that is, for the nth pattern:

$$w_{ij}^{new} = \left(\frac{n-1}{n}\right) w_{ij}^{old} + \left(\frac{1}{n}\right) x_i^{new} x_j^{new}$$

Once the weights have been picked, the memory is ready for operation. It can be visualized as a two-layered network, as shown in Figure 7.3, in which the output at one time becomes the input at the successive time. The input layer is initialized to some state. Next the output of the next layer is computed. This is then used for the input at the next time step. Since the network contains only attractors, the state will evolve to a nearby equilibrium point in the state space.

7.2.1 Stability

How do you show that the network acts like memory? If you were to simulate the network dynamics on a conventional computer, a recourse would be to start from an initial state $x(0)$ and numerically integrate these equations. Fortunately, to analyze what the system does, you don't have to carry out this procedure, as there is a huge insight due to Hopfield[4] that networks with symmetric connections will have no marginally stable states. The states will be either stable or unstable.

Let us try and visualize the state vector x. Extreme values of the state vector form vertices of a hypercube. (A hypercube is an n-dimensional cube. A

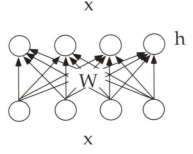

Figure 7.3 The Hopfield network can be visualized as a two-layered network where the output at one time becomes the input at the successive time.

Chapter 7   Content-Addressable Memory

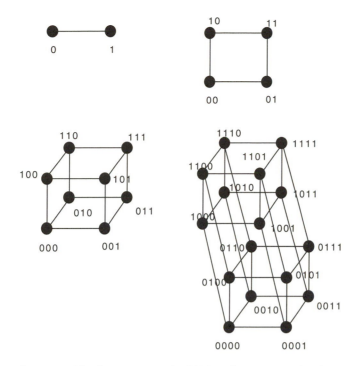

Figure 7.4 The discrete states of a CAM can be represented as the vertices of a hypercube. The codes for each vertex represent a possible state for all the units in the memory. Shown are such cubes for systems of one, two, three, and four states. At any one instant the state is at only one of the vertices.

one-dimensional cube is a line segment, a two-dimensional cube is a square, a three-dimensional cube is a cube, and so forth.) Figure 7.4 shows hypercubes up to four dimensions. To make a fifth-dimensional cube from a fourth, copy the fourth and connect all the corresponding vertices. The state vector is restricted to be a vertex of the cube. Hopfield's insight is that networks that have symmetric weights will have stable states at some of the hypercube vertices. When started at an arbitrary state, the state vector will migrate to one of the vertices and stay there. In contrast, a network without the symmetric weight restriction may oscillate without ever stabilizing.

The symmetric weight criterion allows the derivation of a stability criterion. If the dynamics are allowed to run and the network is stable, it will stabilize at a particular state $\mathbf{x}^p$ such that

$$\mathbf{x}^p = g(W\mathbf{x}^p)$$

or, in terms of the state vector components,

$$x_i^p = g\left(\sum_{j=1}^{N} w_{ij} x_j^p\right) = g(h_i^p)$$

Remember that the weights were set using the Hebb rule, Equation 7.2. This allows the h_i^p term to be written in terms of the stored patterns as

$$h_i^p = \sum_{j=1}^{N} \sum_{q=1}^{Q} x_i^q x_j^q x_j^p$$

Now remove the $p = q$ term, and note also that $x_j^p x_j^p = 1$:

$$h_i^p = N x_i^p + \sum_{j} \sum_{q \neq p} x_i^q x_j^q x_j^p \qquad (7.3)$$

This equation shows that the patterns are stable as long as the second term on the right-hand side is less than N in absolute value. Let us analyze this situation further. Interchanging summations allows the term to be written

$$\sum_{q \neq p} x_i^q \sum_{j} x_j^q x_j^p$$

If the patterns were orthogonal, then

$$x^p \cdot x^q = \sum_{j} x_j^p x_j^q = 0$$

so that the second term would always be guaranteed to be zero. More realistically, though, one might expect that the patterns are chosen randomly. Thus the expected value of the second term is zero, but there will be deviations owing to the variance of the patterns.[5] Since each component of the patterns is either 1 or -1 with equal probability and both the components and the patterns as a whole are independent, then the variance of the "noise" term is just the sum of the variance of each individual term, or

$$\sigma^2 = (Q - 1)N$$

For the usual case of $Q \gg 1$,

$$\sigma^2 = QN$$

Thus, again due to the independence of all the terms in the sum, the variations in this sum will be distributed binomially (Figure 7.5), with mean $\mu = N$ and variance $\sigma^2 = QN$. From this distribution, it is easy to calculate the probability of making an error in an individual bit, as it is the integral under the curve starting from N to ∞, as shown in the figure. Just by inspection, however, one can see that as the number of patterns increases, this ratio will go up, and as the number of units increases, this ratio will go down. But more formally, you can think of the ratio of the mean to the square root of the variance as a signal-to-noise ratio, which is equal to $\sqrt{N/Q}$. When the noise exceeds the signal, there is a probability of making a bit error. The probability of this happening is given by the integral under the normal curve, that is, $\Phi(\frac{-\mu}{\sigma}) = \Phi(\sqrt{N/Q})$. For $N = 1,000$ and $Q = 100$, the probability of making an error is $\Phi(\sqrt{10})$, a very small number indeed.

Another thing to worry about is *storage capacity*. It turns out that the capacity of the CAM is surprisingly low, being approximately $0.138N$.[6]

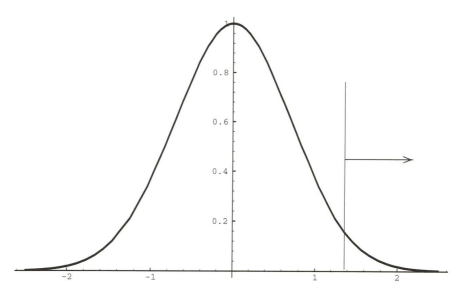

Figure 7.5 The correlation between patterns is binomially distributed. Thus the probability of making an error is just the error under the curve where the noise exceeds the signal. The figure shows the case where $\sqrt{N/Q} = 1.4$.

7.2.2 Lyapunov Stability

The analysis of the previous section is conservative, as it does not take into account the possible beneficial effects of the dynamics of the system. It could be that not all the bits are corrected in one step, but that some of them are, and these help correct additional bits in the next step, and so on. These effects can be analyzed by reconsidering stability. As introduced in Chapter 5, a general result is that if a Lyapunov function $V(x)$ can be found such that $V(x)$ decreases along any trajectory, then the CAM trajectories will always go to local minima. For this case a V that works is the "energy" of the system

$$V = -\frac{1}{2} \sum_i \sum_j w_{ij} x_i x_j$$

Since the diagonal terms contain products $x_i x_i$ that are always 1, these terms can be removed from the summation and written as a constant C. Thus

$$V = C - \sum_{(ij)} w_{ij} x_i x_j$$

where (ij) means distinct pairs; count ij the same as ji. Suppose that x_i' is the next state changed by the update rule. The goal is to show that

$$\Delta V \leq 0$$

that is, that $V(x_i') - V(x_i) \leq 0$. This is trivially true for $x_i' = x_i$, where ΔV is identically 0, so check the case for $x_i' = -x_i$.

$$\Delta V = -\sum_{j \neq i} w_{ij} x_i' x_j + \sum_{j \neq i} w_{ij} x_i x_j$$

$$= 2 \sum_{j \neq i} w_{ij} x_i x_j$$

$$= 2 x_i \sum_j w_{ij} x_j - 2 w_{ii}$$

Now the second term is negative from the Hebb rule, and the first term is negative given the update rule and the assumption that $x_i' = -x_i$. Therefore, $V \leq 0$ along any trajectory. Therefore, all trajectories are stable.

It can also be shown that the memory patterns are local minima.

Another question is the amount that the pattern can be perturbed and still return to its local minimum—in other words the size of its basin of attraction—but this we will leave beyond our scope.

Example: CAM for a Small Phone Book   To make the concept of a content-addressable memory more concrete, consider an experiment by Denker et al.[7] This experiment uses strings of characters from 25-character telephone book entries. The very small database is shown in Figure 7.6.

These entries are encoded into a ± 1 code using five bits per character. For example, a can be encoded as $(-1, -1, -1, -1, 1)$, b as $(-1, -1, -1, 1, -1)$, and so on. Using this strategy, each 25-character entry is encoded as a 125-element pattern vector.

The weights of the network are set by substituting the patterns of bits to be memorized into the Hebb rule. If there are Q patterns x^k, $k = 1,..., Q$ each with n components, then the weights w_{ij} are set according to Equation 7.2. Once these weights are computed the network is ready to be tested.

The experiments show that indeed, starting the network at a state "near" a memory pattern is sufficient to recover the stored pattern, as shown in Figure 7.7. The state of the CAM can be interpreted in terms of characters by using the 5-bit code in reverse. This procedure is followed in the figure, plotting the state of the CAM at regular time intervals. Note the essential property of CAMs that makes them different from standard silicon memories or databases—namely, that the starting key can be arbitrary. Here "john s," the first name and the first letter of the second, is used as the key, but any collection of characters could have been used.

John Stewart Denker	8128
Lawrence David Jackel	7773
Richard Edwin Howard	5952
Wayne P. Hubbard	7707
Brian W. Straughn	3126
John Henry Scofield	8109

Figure 7.6   The database of telephone book entries for the content-addressable memory. (Reprinted from *Physica D: Nonlinear Phenomena*, 22D[1–3], John S. Denker, "Neural Models of Learning and Adaptation," pp. 216–32, © 1986 with kind permission of Elsevier Science—NL, Sara Burgerhartstraat 25, 1055 KV Amsterdam, The Netherlands.)

Time	Energy	CAM state
0.0	0.0	john s
0.2	-0.0784	john sdewirubneoimv 8109
0.4	-0.8426	john sdewirtbnenimv 8129
0.6	-0.8451	john sdewirtbnenimv 8129
0.8	-0.8581	john sdewirt nenkmv 8128
1.0	-0.9099	john sdewart denker 8128
1.2	-0.9824	john stewart denker 8128

Figure 7.7 Results of using the CAM. The basic feature of content-addressable memory is illustrated: items are recoverable regardless of the form of the "key." Also shown are the values for *V*. (Reprinted from *Physica D: Nonlinear Phenomena,* 22D[1–3], John S. Denker, "Neural Models of Learning and Adaptation," pp. 216–32, © 1986 with kind permission of Elsevier Science–NL, Sara Burgerhartstraat 25, 1055 KV Amsterdam, The Netherlands.)

Time	Energy	CAM state
0.0	0.0	garbage
0.2	-0.0244	garbagee lafj naabd 5173
0.4	-0.6280	garbaged derjd naabd 7173
0.6	-0.6904	garbaged derjd naabd 7173
0.8	-0.6904	gasbafed derjd naabd 7173
1.0	-0.7595	gasbabed derjd naabd 7173
1.2	-0.7709	fasjebad derjd naabd 7173
1.4	-0.8276	fasjebad derjd naabd 7173
1.6	-0.8282	fasjeb d derjd naabd 7173

Figure 7.8 Results of starting from a point in state space that is not near any of the memories. The dynamics takes the state to a local minimum that is not a stored item. (Reprinted from *Physica D: Nonlinear Phenomena,* 22D[1–3], John S. Denker, "Neural Models of Learning and Adaptation," pp. 216–32, © 1986 with kind permission of Elsevier Science–NL, Sara Burgerhartstraat 25, 1055 KV Amsterdam, The Netherlands.)

The value of the energy, *V,* is also shown. Note that, as expected in a gradient search strategy, the value for *V* is monotonically decreasing.

Figure 7.8 also shows an undesirable property of the Hopfield CAM: there are spurious local minima. If the state is started sufficiently far from a memory, the resultant attractor may not be a memory, but may be one of these other local minima.[8]

7.3 KANERVA MEMORIES

Consider storing Q memories using n bits where $Q \ll 2^n$. Further, consider that the memories are uncorrelated. These assumptions mean that the memories are both *sparse* and *distributed.* These two properties are essential for the Kanerva memories, which are sometimes also referred to as sparse, distributed memories. Kanerva memories can also be heteroassociative. Pairs of data (x, y) are to be stored and retrieved. It turns out that an unusual strategy works. Pick M data vectors that are sparsely distributed in the memory. Next, for the vector to be stored, x, add its contents y to all the vectors d that are within Hamming distance D of x. To recover the vector, find the data vectors by the same procedure, add them, and threshold their contents; that is,

$$y_i = g\left(\sum d_i\right)$$

This strategy is illustrated in abstract form in Figure 7.9, which shows three memory locations (closed circles) that are within D of the item to be recovered or stored (open circle).

You can see that if a single vector were treated this way it would be recovered correctly. Copies of the data would be retrieved from nearby locations. Their sums when thresholded would yield the original data vector. What happens in the general case of many vectors is that the contents of a data vector may reflect the sum of more than one input vector. However, as values of the vector's individual components are ± 1 and they are assumed to be randomly distributed, the effects of the components from other vectors tend to cancel, and the sums of the copies of the input vector predominate.

To make this idea even more concrete, it will be helpful to compare this scheme to conventional computer memory. A conventional computer memory uses a dense address space. For example, with 20 bits of address space, all 2^{20} locations are used. To access a location, the location's address is selected, and the contents are modified, as shown in Figure 7.10. In contrast, Kanerva memory uses a sparse address space of locations that have considerably more bits than conventional memory. For exam-

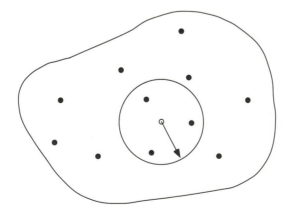

Figure 7.9 An abstraction of the Kanerva memory scheme illustrates the basic idea. Memory locations are sparsely distributed within the address space. A given memory is stored redundantly at all the locations within distance D. To retrieve the memory, these locations are found and their contents added and thresholded.

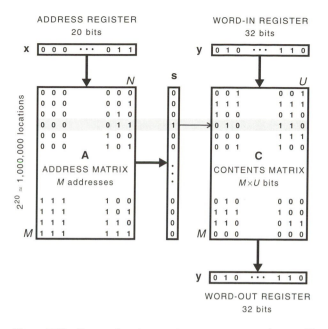

Figure 7.10 Conventional computer memory uses a dense address space. To access a location, the location's address is selected and the contents written or read. (From Kanerva, 1993; © 1993 by Pentti Kanerva and used with his permission.)

ple, 1,000-bit addresses would not be unusual. However, there is no way of having $2^{1,000}$ physical memory locations! As shown in Figure 7.11, accessing a memory involves finding all the sparse locations that are within a distance D of the address. The contents of these vectors are then summed and thresholded.[9]

7.3.1 Implementation

The formal specification of the Kanerva strategy uses two matrices, one for the addresses and one for the contents. Let us call them A and C, respectively. The first thing to do is calculate the set of data vectors that are close to the input x. If the $M \times N$ matrix A is used to hold the addresses, the distances between x and the addresses can be expressed as Ax. Let the ones that are within a distance D be represented by a *select* vector s. Then

$$s = \Theta_D(Ax)$$

where Θ_D is the threshold function that uses Hamming distance D. In other words, s is M units long and has an entry of 1 at a given position if the corresponding row of A is within D units of x.

The distance D determines the number of ones in the select vector, which corresponds to the number of nearby memories. For the memory to work best, the number of neighbors should be chosen so that there are a fraction p of them, so that a fraction pM of the memory items are within D units of the item. The fraction pM should be not too large or too small. We

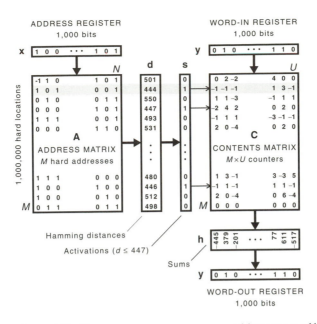

Figure 7.11 Kanerva memory uses a sparse address space of locations that have considerably more bits than conventional memory. When storing a pattern, all the nearby address locations are selected and the contents summed with the current contents at each of those locations. To retrieve a pattern, the locations are accessed as before, and the contents of each of those locations are summed and thresholded. The address space may be represented as a matrix *A*, and the contents as a matrix *C*. (From Kanerva, 1993; © 1993 by Pentti Kanerva and used with his permission.)

will return to this point when we analyze the performance of the memories; for now just assume that the best p is used.

The next step is to add the contents of the vector to each of the selected prototypes. This is done by

$$C = \sum_{k=1}^{Q} s^k \left(y^k \right)^T \tag{7.4}$$

(If you check this out with just one pattern, you will see that the formula adds in the pattern in all the right places in the *C* matrix.)

Once the vectors have been stored in this way, getting the contents of a particular one back is easy. First the select vector accesses the appropriate elements of the data matrix *C*:

$$h = s^T C$$

Then h is thresholded to produce the pattern

$$y = g(h)$$

where $g()$ is a *vector* threshold function

$$g_i(x) = \begin{cases} +1 & x_i \geq 0 \\ -1 & \text{otherwise} \end{cases}$$

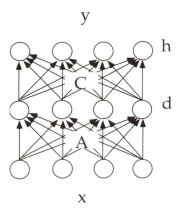

y

h

d

x

Figure 7.12   Kanerva memory can be implemented in a three-layered network.

These operations can be thought of as implemented in a three-layered network, as shown in Figure 7.12. The first layer contains the A matrix as weights. Each row of the A matrix can be thought of as the receptive field of a unit, and there are M units total. The units at the second layer are then thresholded with a threshold D to produce the vector s. The second layer contains the C matrix. Each column of the C matrix can be thought of as the receptive field of a unit in the last layer. Thus the input to this layer is the sums of all the appropriate C matrix columns, which are then thresholded for the answer.

7.3.2   Performance of Kanerva Memories

If the memory works well, when the system is presented with input x it will produce the associated vector y. Let us explore the conditions under which that outcome occurs. Denote a particular input pattern as x^a, so that

$$s^a = \Theta_D(Ax^a)$$

Then using Equation 7.4, h is given by

$$h = s^a \sum_{k=1}^{Q} s^k \left(y^k\right)^T \tag{7.5}$$

In the Hopfield memories, the analogous equation (Equation 7.3) was separated into a data term and a noise term. The same technique can be used here to break Equation 7.5 into a data term and a noise term.

$$h = y^a \left(s^a \cdot s^a\right) + \sum_{k=1, k \neq a}^{Q} s^a s^k \left(y^k\right)^T \tag{7.6}$$

Remember that the memory was set up to have on the order of pM ones in the select vector where $p \ll 1$. Thus the expected value of the first term is pMy^a and, of course, $y^a = g(pMy^a)$. Thus whether or not the vector is recovered depends again on the variance. If the basis vectors are randomly chosen, the noise can be calculated as follows. Let

$$L_k = s^{kT} \cdot s^k$$

and consider the case of the ith bit in the memory. Assume that this is 1 (the case of -1 is handled the same way).

$$\sigma^2 = \text{var}\left[y_i^a\left(s^a \cdot s^a\right) + \sum_{k=1, k \neq a}^{Q} y_i^k s^{kT} s^k \right]$$

$$= \text{var}(L_a) + \text{var}\left(\sum_{k=1, k \neq a}^{Q} y_i^k s^k \cdot s^k \right)$$

Assuming the individual terms in the sum are independent allows this equation to be written as

$$= \text{var}(L_a) + (Q - 1)\text{var}(y_1 L_1)$$

The variance of the first term is approximately pM. Now consider just the variance of the second term without the multiplier $Q - 1$. This can be expressed as

$$E(y_1^2 L_1^2) - E(y_1 L_1)^2$$

but the last term is just 0, and the first term is just $E(L_1^2)$, so it can now be expressed in terms of variance as

$$\text{var}(L_1) + E(L_1)^2$$

The probability of the sum at any particular memory location can be modeled as a Poisson distribution with parameter pM, that is, $p(L) = pM^x e^{-pM}/L!$. As a consequence, the mean is p^2M and the variance is also p^2M. Thus the expression for σ^2 becomes, finally,

$$\sigma^2 = pM + (Q - 1)[p^2M + (p^2M)^2]$$

When Q is much larger than 1, this can be written as

$$\sigma^2 = pM[1 + pQ(1 + p^2M)]$$

This has been a lengthy derivation, but it is not without reward. You can now calculate the probability that the memory works correctly, that is, that a bit will be recalled without error. Assuming all the components of the sum to be independent allows them to be approximated with a normal distribution of mean μ and variance σ^2. The probability that the ith bit will be in error is simply the probability that its sum, h_i, is less than zero (remember that we assumed that the bit was one). Using the assumption of a normal distribution is simply

$$\Phi(-\mu/\sigma)$$

where $\mu = pM$ and σ is given previously.

Example of a Kanerva Memory   For a given memory

$$Q = 100, p = .01, \text{ and } M = 10,000$$

Then

$$\mu = 100 \text{ and } \sigma = \sqrt{100[1 + 1(1 + 1)]} = 10\sqrt{3}$$

so that the probability of an error is $\Phi(5.77)$.

7.3.3 Implementations of Kanerva Memories

To make these ideas clear, consider two examples from Kanerva.

The first example shows the CAM feature. Figure 7.13 shows nine memory vectors that are defined on a 256-bit memory space. The 16×16 pictorial format allows you to see that they are close to each other, as they share many elements in common. Into this memory a circle is stored. The circle will be near each of the memories, and its bits will be included in their internal sums of the C matrix. The bottom part of the figure shows the process of recovering the stored memory from a more distant starting point. When the bit pattern on the left is entered, the middle pattern is retrieved. When that is used as an index to the memory, the rightmost pattern is retrieved, and that is a stable pattern.

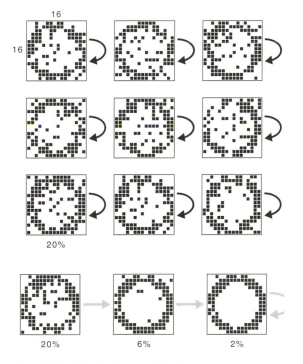

Figure 7.13 The black and white dots each represent a component of the memory and are encoded as ± 1. (*upper*) Nine memory vectors are defined on a 256-bit memory space that is represented in a 16×16 pictorial format for ease of visualization. The arrows indicate that these are stable patterns. Into this memory a circle is stored. (*lower*) Retrieving the stored memory. When the bit pattern on the left is entered, the middle pattern is retrieved. When that is used as an index to the memory, the rightmost pattern is retrieved, and that is a stable pattern. (From Kanerva, 1993; © 1993 by Pentti Kanerva and used with his permission.)

The second example shows the heteroassociative feature of Kanerva memories. When the length of the pattern and address are equal, this fact allows for the storage of pattern sequences. In this case the sequence $x^1, x^2, x^3,\ldots, x^k$ can be stored by converting the sequence into pairwise associations:

$$x^1, x^2$$
$$x^2, x^3$$
$$\vdots$$
$$x^{k-1}, x^k$$

In other words, the content of pattern one is pattern two, which in turn is an address with pattern three as its contents. Starting the memory with pattern one allows the recovery of pattern two, and so on. Figure 7.14 shows another example of using patterns that have a pictorial interpretation. In this case sequences of Roman numeral "images" are associated. The figure shows the response of the memory when starting from the point of a distorted "three." Given this point, the rest of the sequence is recovered.

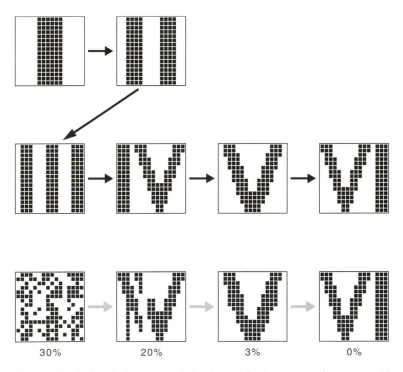

Figure 7.14 Using the heteroassociative feature for the storage of sequences. The content of pattern one is pattern two, which in turn is an address with pattern three as its contents. Starting the memory close to pattern three allows the rest of the sequence to be recovered. Percentages indicate the bits in error in each pattern. (From Kanerva, 1993; © 1993 by Pentti Kanerva and used with his permission.)

7.4 RADIAL BASIS FUNCTIONS

The essential idea of Kanerva memories is illustrated in Figure 7.9. Information is stored in multiple nearby locations in multidimensional space. The redundant storage allows it to be recovered with extremely low error rates. Although the value stored was related to the memory address by being a point in the same representational space, you could have just as easily stored a number related to a *function* of that address. In this view the Kanerva memory can be seen as doing function approximation. A coefficient is known at the "hard" or physical memory locations, and can be used to recover the function values by interpolation.

A useful form of the functions for this interpolation is a form of a general class of functions called *radial basis functions*. The general form is that the response of a specific point x_i can be written as

$$h(x) = g(\|x - x_i\|)$$

The specific function we used before was the threshold function

$$h(x) = 1 \text{ if hamming\_dist } (x, x_i) < D$$

but another example would be a Gaussian:

$$h_i(x) = e^{\frac{-(\|x-x_i\|^2)}{2\sigma_i^2}}$$

Now suppose that the problem is to recover a specific function of $f(x)$ rather than x itself. A way to do this would be to interpolate values of f using coefficients c_i stored at nearby locations using the radial basis functions. In other words,

$$f(x) = \sum_i c_i h_i(x) \tag{7.7}$$

If there are M values of f, then Equation 7.7 represents a linear set of m equations in M unknowns that can be solved for the c provided the matrix $W = w_{ij}$ represented by $h_i(x_j)$ is invertible. It turns out that in most cases it is.

Solving Equation 7.7 will get the values right for the specific points x_i, but getting the function values right for x between these points is another matter, and this depends on the values of σ_i. Herein we will be content with determining a best value in the case $\sigma_i = \sigma_0$, $i = 1,..., N$ (see exercises).[10]

7.5 KALMAN FILTERING

Yet another extension to Kanerva memories is that of combating the effects of noise. Remember from the example at the end of Chapter 3 that it was possible to think of the job of the memory as representing a compact code for the input. Starting from the idea of minimizing the cost of the model plus the cost of the data described with the model motivated the use of the objective function

$$E(W, x) = a\|W\|^2 + \beta\|x\|^2 + \|I - Wx\|^2$$

where I was the input image, x the responses of a set of units, and W a matrix of weights connecting the input to these units. Differentiating with respect to x and using gradient descent provides a dynamics for the units:

$$\dot{x} = -\frac{\eta}{2}\frac{\partial E}{\partial x} = -k_1 x + k_2 W^T(I - Wx)$$

Now assume that this equation is corrupted by having noise μ added:

$$\dot{x} = -k_1 x + k_2 W^T(I - Wx) + \mu$$

where μ has parameters

$$E[\mu] = 0 \text{ and } E[\mu\mu^T] = Q$$

Let's also assume that there is an internal estimate of x, which we will call $\bar{x}$. This is assumed to be related to the internal value by a measurement equation

$$\bar{x} = x + v$$

where v is a noise vector with parameters

$$E[\mu] = 0 \text{ and } E[vv^T] = R$$

The solution to this problem was previously developed in Chapter 6 and is the Kalman filter. Making the appropriate identifications,[11]

$$\dot{\hat{x}} = -k_1 x + k_2 W^T(I - Wx) + PR^{-1}(\bar{x} - \hat{x})$$

where P is the covariance matrix for the error $(x - \hat{x})$ and must be computed iteratively, as discussed in Chapter 6.

NOTES

1. This is a controversial assumption because the synapses of a neuron could also be used as memory units; e.g., Bartlett W. Mel, "Information Processing in Dendritic Trees," *Neural Computation* 6, no. 6 (Nov. 1, 1994):1031.

2. Real neurons can represent negative numbers in at least two different ways. One is to have a baseline firing rate mean "zero." Another is to use two neurons to represent the signal, one for the positive part and one for the negative part.

3. This rule is named after Donald Hebb, who first suggested that synaptic strengths might be determined by the correlation between pre- and postsynaptic neural firing patterns.

4. J. Hopfield, "Neural Networks and Physical Systems with Emergent Collective Computational Abilities," *Proceedings of the National Academy of Sciences, USA* 79 (1982):2554–58.

5. The analysis of the variance here and with respect to Kanerva memories is due to a beautiful paper by J. D. Keeler entitled "Comparison Between Kanerva's SDM and Hopfield-Type Neural Networks," *Cognitive Science* 12 (1988):299–329.

6. The proof of this statement is very involved, and will be found in an advanced text such as *Introduction to the Theory of Neural Computation* (Lecture Notes Volume 1, Santa Fe Institute Studies in the Sciences of Complexity) by John Hertz, Anders Krogh, and Richard G. Palmer (Redwood City, CA: Addison-Wesley, 1991).

7. John S. Denker, "Neural Models of Learning and Adaptation," *Physica D: Nonlinear Phenomena*, 22D, no. 1–3 (Oct.–Nov. 1986):216–32.

8. The properties of these minima have been extensively analyzed, e.g., in D. Amit, H. Gutfreund, and H. Sompolinsky, "Spin-Glass Models of Neural Networks," *Physical Review A* 32 (1985):1007–18.

9. P. Kanerva, "Sparse Distributed Memory and Related Models," in Mohamad H. Hassoun, ed., *Associative Neural Memories: Theory and Implementation* (New York: Oxford University Press, 1993, pp. 50–76).

10. An excellent review of the various methods for finding these values is contained in *Neural Networks for Pattern Recognition* by Christopher M. Bishop (New York: Oxford University Press, 1995).

11. R. N. Rao and D. H. Ballard, *Dynamic Model of Visual Memory Predicts Neural Response Properties in the Visual Cortex*, NRL Tech. Report 95.4, Department of Computer Science, University of Rochester, N.Y., 1995.

EXERCISES

1. Show that memory patterns are local minima.

2. Assume a continuous activation function of the form $g(x) = \frac{1}{1 + e^{-x}}$ and show that $H(x) = -x^T W x$ is a Lyapunov function for the system.

3. Build a Hopfield content-addressable memory and run experiments to test its capacity. Use a five-bit code for letters and numbers. Each memory item should take 125 bits and encode name, abbreviated address, and university extension. Specific functionality:

• Implement functions *add-an-entry* and *delete-an-entry*.
• Demonstrate a false match by picking the right basin of attraction.
• Demonstrate the capacity by plotting the number of successful retrievals from random starting points as a function of (a) the percent of the entry used in the initial condition and (b) the number of entries in memory.

4. Your job is to build a Kanerva memory using the physical memory addresses

$$x^1 = \begin{pmatrix} -1 \\ 1 \\ -1 \\ 1 \\ 1 \end{pmatrix}, x^2 = \begin{pmatrix} 1 \\ -1 \\ 1 \\ 1 \\ 1 \end{pmatrix}, x^3 = \begin{pmatrix} -1 \\ -1 \\ 1 \\ -1 \\ -1 \end{pmatrix}, x^4 = \begin{pmatrix} 1 \\ -1 \\ -1 \\ -1 \\ 1 \end{pmatrix}$$

Show how, using a threshold of 2, you would store the items

$$\begin{pmatrix} 1 \\ 1 \\ -1 \\ 1 \\ 1 \end{pmatrix} \text{ and } \begin{pmatrix} -1 \\ -1 \\ -1 \\ -1 \\ -1 \end{pmatrix}$$

5. Calculate the probability of an error in a Kanerva memory when the number of items is $Q = 500$, the probability of storing a memory at a location is $p = .05$, and the number of memories is $M = 5,000$.

6. In a Kanerva memory the number of points within a distance D of an arbitrary point can be calculated by a binomial distribution:

$$N(D) = \frac{\sum_{k=0}^{D} \frac{n!}{(n - k)!k!}}{2^n}$$

Approximate this with a normal distribution and comment on the behavior of the distribution for increasing n.

7. From the formula for calculating the probability of a bit error, $\Phi(\frac{-\mu}{\sigma})$, it is clear that the larger the ratio $\rho = \mu/\sigma$, the better. Use this observation to find the optimum value of p in terms of Q and M by finding the p that maximizes ρ^2.

8. In the example of using the Kalman filter, the idea was to construct an internal image $I' = Wx$ that approximates the input image as closely as possible. Suppose you allow the internal image to have a first-order term using a Taylor series expansion in terms of a spatial variable y, so that

$$I = I' + \frac{\partial I'}{\partial y} \Delta y$$

Show how you would extend the Kalman filter model to handle this case.

9. Suggest how the formalism of Exercise 8 could be used to model the case of stereo input images. (See R. N. Rao and D. H. Ballard, *A Class of Stochastic Models for Invariant Recognition, Motion, and Stereo*, NRL Tech. Report 96.1, Department of Computer Science, University of Rochester, N.Y., 1996.)

10. Approximate the function $y(x) = \sin(x)$ in the interval $[0, 2\pi]$ with 16 radial basis functions. Determine by experiment the value of σ that best represents the data.

8 Supervised Learning

ABSTRACT   A special property of memories is that they should generalize the patterns that they store. Thus, in a heteroassociative memory, if a pattern x appears that is like a stored pattern x_0 that is associated with y_0, the desired response should be appropriately similar to y_0. To apply this principle in a general way requires a new kind of algorithm that is introduced here. This algorithm uses additional units that allow very nonlinear generalizations. The algorithm works on a layered, feedforward network, but under certain circumstances, recurrent networks can be modeled as layered feedforward networks. The complexity of the generalizations is related to the number of layers in the network.

8.1   INTRODUCTION

A central idea of the content-addressable memory is that of the attractor state. If an input is close to a memory, the dynamics of the system as captured by the weights will drive the state of the system to the nearby memory. The region near the memory for which this process works is called its *basin of attraction*. This works well when variations in the stored patterns are clumped near their attractors, but less well when the pattern variations overlap each other in the state space. In the latter case, the patterns can extend beyond the basin of attraction. Figure 8.1 shows such a case.

   Ideally what one would like to do is have control over the shape of the basin of attraction for each memory. However, since the units of the CAM are notionally input units, there are no degrees of freedom left to sculpt the basin of attraction. To do so requires additional units that are not directly inputs or outputs of the system. For that reason they are called *hidden units*. With such units one can realize the goal of creating arbitrarily shaped basins of attraction. Another way to think of this process is to regard the associated pattern as the *classification* of the input pattern. A second goal is to speed up the process of computing an output. If you think of the network as a heteroassociative memory, you might also like the memory to compute the associated pattern or classification in one "step." This chapter shows how to design such networks that accomplish both goals. The networks that do so are *feedforward* networks. Such networks have no cycles; that is, there is no path from any unit leading back to itself. Layered feedforward networks have their units organized in layers and further restrict the connections to just those units at the subsequent layer.

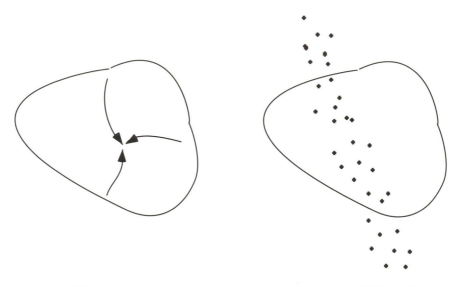

Figure 8.1 (*left*) A basin of attraction for a given memory state vector. (*right*) The motivating problem: points that are notionally the same prototype are not all included in the basin of attraction.

The networks that shape the classification boundaries must have multiple layers. Early experiments with single-layered networks caused much excitement until it was proved that such networks were limited to linear separation boundaries. Such networks were termed *perceptrons* by their creator, Frank Rosenblatt.[1] The extensions to multilayered networks removed this limitation.

The restriction to layered feedforward networks may seem severe, but that turns out not to be the case at all. Generally connected or *recurrent networks* can be modeled as layered feedforward networks by a process of "unrolling" the computations in time.

8.2 PERCEPTRONS

The perceptron is illustrated in Figure 8.2 (*top*). Even though the properties of multilayered networks are our goal, the perceptron is a good place to start. The study of perceptrons lends itself to an elucidation of the geometry associated with the accompanying learning algorithms. In particular, one can show how single-layered networks are limited to linear separation surfaces, a limiting property that is not present with multilayered networks.

Like Hopfield memories, a perceptron's output y_i is determined by

$$y_i = g\left(\sum_k w_{ik} x_k\right)$$

where $g(h) = \text{sgn}\,(h)$, that is, the sign of h. The *classification problem* is to adjust the weights so that $y_i = y_i^d$. Now since the output units are independent of each other, just look at the value of any particular unit. Thus the subscript i can be dropped (see Figure 8.2, *bottom*).

Chapter 8   Supervised Learning

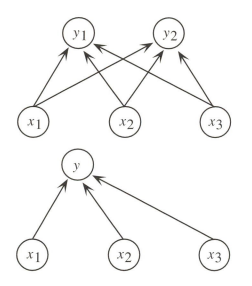

Figure 8.2 (*top*) The perceptron is a single-layered, feedforward network in which the output of each unit is determined by a threshold function. (*bottom*) Since each output unit is independent of the others, its behavior can be analyzed separately.

In the simplest case, $y_i^d = \pm 1$. Thus we want

$$\text{sgn}(\mathbf{w} \cdot \mathbf{x}^p) = y^p$$

This criterion can be satisfied if there is a line that separates the members of the two classes; in other words, if they are *linearly separable,* as shown in the top part of Figure 8.3. In three dimensions the surface will be a plane, and in the general case of a many-dimensional state space, the separating surface will be a hyperplane.

A final simplification occurs with the change of variables,

$$\mathbf{z}^p = y^p \mathbf{x}^p \tag{8.1}$$

so that now the criterion for separability becomes

$$\mathbf{w} \cdot \mathbf{z}^p > 0$$

This transformation is shown in the lower part of Figure 8.3, which makes the obvious but crucial point that to work without error, all the transformed points must lie in a half-plane, and thus the original data must have been linearly separable.

The transformation of Equation 8.1 works for problems for which the separating surface goes through the origin. What happens when the surface cannot? Logical OR is a case in point. For this problem the desired associations are shown in Table 8.1. This can always be converted to the original problem by adding a threshold, as shown in Figure 8.4. A threshold can in turn be thought of as an extra input with value -1 and weight w_{io}.

Perceptron Learning Rule   For a particular pattern p we want the condition $\mathbf{w} \cdot \mathbf{z}^p > 0$ to hold. Suppose that it does not. Let us change $\mathbf{w}$ by an amount $-(\mathbf{w} \cdot \mathbf{z}^p)\mathbf{z}^p$. To interpret this expression, observe that $(\mathbf{w} \cdot \mathbf{z}^p)$ is

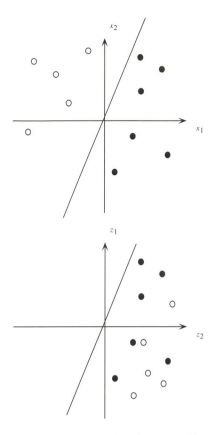

Figure 8.3 (*top*) The classification problem with linearly separable patterns. (*bottom*) Changing variables transforms the problem into one of placing all the points on the same side of a plane.

Table 8.1 The patterns that represent OR.

$x_1 x_2$	y
0 0	0
0 1	1
1 0	1
1 1	1

the projection of w onto z^p. If this is positive, then the condition is met. Otherwise, add a little of the vector z^p to w. This addition moves w closer into alignment with z^p and makes the projection more positive.

This reasoning leads directly to a simplified[2] version of the *perceptron learning rule:*

$$\Delta w = -\eta \Theta[w \cdot z^p] z^p$$

where

$$\Theta[x] = \begin{cases} 1 & \text{if } x > 0 \\ 0 & \text{otherwise} \end{cases}$$

The effect of this rule is illustrated in Figure 8.5.

Chapter 8 Supervised Learning

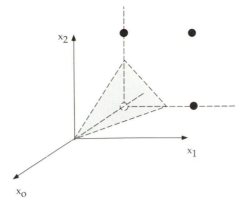

Figure 8.4 Adding a threshold allows the separation surface to go through the origin in the higher-dimensional space. In the three-dimensional space shown, all the input vectors have their x_0 component equal to -1. The extra degree of freedom in the weight vector allows the plane to be tilted to separate the classes.

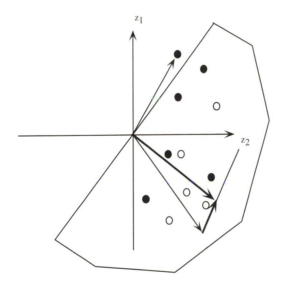

Figure 8.5 The perceptron learning rule: If a pattern is misclassified, its projection onto the weight vector is proportional to the weight vector correction.

8.3 CONTINUOUS ACTIVATION FUNCTIONS

The perceptron captures many of the basic intuitions that surround the problem of separating data in a vector space. Its weakness turns out to be the use of a threshold activation function. Deciding how to handle the weight updates in multilayered networks turns on a continuous activation function, as this allows the modeling of the different inter-network variable dependencies with derivatives.

Continuous activation functions were introduced with the Widrow-Hoff learning rule in Chapter 6. They allow the adjustment of the weights

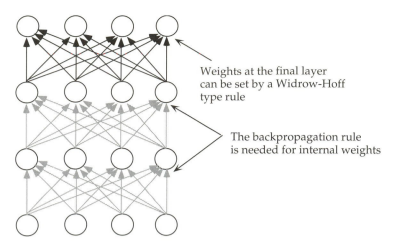

Weights at the final layer
can be set by a Widrow-Hoff
type rule

The backpropagation rule
is needed for internal weights

Figure 8.6 The problem for multilayered networks is to adjust the internal weights. The solution is to derive a relationship between the error correction of the final layer and the error correction at earlier layers. As this rule passes the correction backward through the network, it is known as backpropagation.

to the output layer. This adjustment is easy to make because the effect of the weights on the output units is easily calculated. But the situation is more complicated for multilayered networks, as shown in Figure 8.6, because the weights to internal units must be adjusted and their effects are indirect: They affect only the outputs of internal units, which in turn affect the output units.

The Widrow-Hoff formulation is on track in a crucial way in that, since the activation function is differentiable, the techniques of optimization theory can be used. However, a linear activation function does not add anything to a multilayered feedforward network, as such a network can always be reduced to an equivalent single-layered network. To extend the network properties, the activation function must be nonlinear. The nonlinear differentiable function that we will use is inspired by neurons that have saturating firing rates; it is shown in Figure 8.7.

To keep things simple, let us just work with one pattern. In that case the objective function is defined to be

$$E = \frac{1}{2}\|x^K - d\|^2 \tag{8.2}$$

where K is an index denoting the last layer in the network and d is the desired output.

The equation for updating the states is given by

$$x^{k+1} = g(W^k x^k) \tag{8.3}$$

where W^k is a matrix used to store the weights between layer k and layer $k + 1$,

$$W^k = \begin{bmatrix} w^k_{11} & w^k_{12} & \cdots \\ w^k_{21} & & \ddots \\ \vdots & & w^k_{nn} \end{bmatrix} = \begin{pmatrix} w^k_1 \\ w^k_2 \\ \vdots \\ w^k_n \end{pmatrix}$$

and the special understanding we shall have is that the function g applied to a vector is just that function applied to its elements; that is,

$$g(Wx) = \begin{pmatrix} g(w_1 \cdot x) \\ g(w_2 \cdot x) \\ \vdots \end{pmatrix}$$

Do you see that you have encountered this problem before? This is just a version of the optimal control problem introduced in Chapter 6 where Equation 8.2 is the optimand and Equation 8.3 is the dynamics. Here instead of the control u, the matrices W^k, $k = 1,\ldots, K$ represent the "control" variables. One difference, of course, is the dimensionality. In the cart problem in Chapter 6, for example, the state space was only two-dimensional. In networks the dimension of the state space may range into the thousands! But the important thing to realize is that the mathematical treatment is the same.

Thus this problem can be tackled using the Euler-Lagrange formulation. The Hamiltonian is defined to be

$$H = \frac{1}{2} \|x^K - d\|^2 + \sum_{k=0}^{k=K-1} (\lambda^{k+1})^T [-x^{k+1} + g(W^k x^k)]$$

where the first term measures the cost of errors reproducing the pattern and the second term constrains the system to follow its dynamic

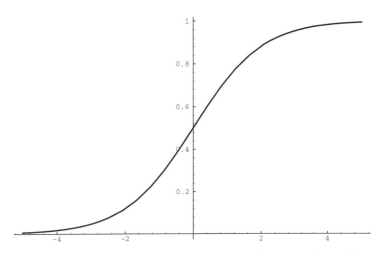

Figure 8.7 The nonlinear differentiable activation function used in multilayered networks.

8.3 Continuous Activation Functions

equations. Differentiating with respect to x^k provides the adjoint system of equations,

$$H_{x^k} = 0 = -\lambda^k + [W^{kT}\Lambda^{k+1}g'(W^k x^k)] \text{ for } k = 0,\ldots, K - 1 \qquad (8.4)$$

where

$$\Lambda^{k+1} = \begin{bmatrix} \lambda_1^{k+1} & 0 & \cdots \\ 0 & \lambda_2^{k+1} & \\ \vdots & & \lambda_n^{k+1} \end{bmatrix}$$

and with the final condition given by

$$H_{x^K} = 0 = x^K - d - \lambda^K \text{ for } k = K$$

8.3.1 Unpacking the Notation

To understand Equation 8.4, consider the case where the number of units in each layer is just two. Then

$$(\lambda^{k+1})^T g(W^k x^k) = \lambda_1^{k+1} g(w_{11}x_1^k + w_{12}x_2^k) + \lambda_2^{k+1} g(w_{21}x_1^k + w_{22}x_2^k)$$

Taking the partial derivative with respect to x_1^k,

$$\lambda_1^{k+1} g'(w_{11}x_1^k + w_{12}x_2^k)w_{11} + \lambda_2^{k+1} g'(w_{21}x_1^k + w_{22}x_2^k)w_{21}$$

Similarly the partial derivative with respect to x_2^k,

$$\lambda_1^{k+1} g'(w_{11}x_1^k + w_{12}x_2^k)w_{12} + \lambda_2^{k+1} g'(w_{21}x_1^k + w_{22}x_2^k)w_{22}$$

Reassembling these terms into a vector results in

$$W^{kT} \begin{pmatrix} \lambda_1^{k+1} g'(w_1^k \cdot x^k) \\ \lambda_2^{k+1} g'(w_2^k \cdot x^k) \\ \vdots \end{pmatrix} = W^{kT}\Lambda^{k+1}g'(W^k x^k)$$

8.3.2 Generating the Solution

To generate the solution, assume an initial W matrix. Then solve the dynamic equations going forward in levels in the network. This solution provides a value for x^K. This value allows the adjoint system to be solved backward for $k = K$ to $k = 0$:

$$\lambda^K = x^K - d \text{ for } k = K$$

$$\lambda^k = W^{kT}\Lambda^{k+1}g'(W^k x^k) \text{ for } k = 0,\ldots, K - 1$$

where g' denotes differentiation with respect to its argument. Now improve the estimate for W using gradient descent. To do so, calculate the adjustment for the weights as $\frac{\partial H}{\partial w_{ij}}$:

$$\frac{\partial H}{\partial w_{ij}^k} = \lambda_i^{k+1} x_j^k g'(w_i^k \cdot x^k) \tag{8.5}$$

Equation 8.5 is very compact and so is worth unpacking in order to understand it. The multiplier λ_i^{k+1} can be understood by realizing that at level K it just keeps track of the output error. This is its role for the internal units also; it appropriately keeps track of how the internal weight change affects output error. The derivative g' is also simple, especially when using

$$g(u) = \frac{1}{1 + e^{-u}}$$

since it can be easily verified that

$$g'(u) = g(1 - g)$$

Thus to calculate g' for a given unit, just determine how much input the x_j^kth unit receives, and apply that as an argument to $g'()$.

Putting all this together results in Algorithm 8.1.[3]

Algorithm 8.1   Backpropagation

Until the error is sufficiently small, do the following for each pattern:

1. Apply the pattern to the network and calculate the state variables using Equation 8.3.

2. Solve the adjoint Equation 8.4.

3. Adjust the weights W^k using

$$\Delta w_{ij}^k = -\eta \frac{\partial H}{\partial w_{ij}^k}$$

where $\frac{\partial H}{\partial w_{ij}^k}$ is given by Equation 8.5.

Notice the change in the formulation in the backpropagation equations. The original problem in Chapter 6 was formulated with time as a dependent variable. Translating to the network formulation, the dependent variable became the different hidden state variables in the network. Time was translated into space.

In developing this algorithm only one pattern was used, but the extension to multiple patterns is straightforward. The strictly correct thing to do would be to accumulate the weight changes for each pattern separately, add them up, and then adjust the weight vector accordingly. The problem with this approach is that the calculations for each pattern are laborious. To make faster progress one can approximate the strict method by adjusting the weights after each pattern is used. This technique is known as *stochastic gradient descent*. The understanding is that the sum of the successive corrections should approximate the sum of all the corrections that are computed simultaneously.

Example: Learning Family Trees   As an example of the backpropagation algorithm in action, consider the following example from Rumelhart et al.[4] The task of the network is to learn family relationships. The database of relationships comes from two isomorphic family trees, one English and one Italian, which are shown in Figure 8.8.

The network has four layers, as shown in Figure 8.9. To train the network, triples of (*person, relationship, relation*) are used, such as (*Alfonso, father, Marco*). The appropriate units are turned on in the network, and the measured error is propagated using the backpropagation algorithm. Only a subset of the relationships is used in training.

To test the network, the first two elements of a triplet are applied to the input units. For example, the input (*Colin, aunt*) is represented by turning on the appropriate two units representing the person and the relationship, as shown in Figure 8.10. The units that are turned on the most in the output bank of units represent the answer. In this case the output shows that the two units most activated represent Colin's aunts, the correct answer.

The most interesting aspect of the multilayered networks is the hidden units. It has been shown in experiment after experiment that these units evolve into compact codes for parts of the patterns. This hidden unit property is true also for the family tree example. The best way to see it is to look at the weights for individual units, as these weights determine their responses. Let us look at the weights for two hidden units in the second layer of the family tree network that are connected to the input person units.

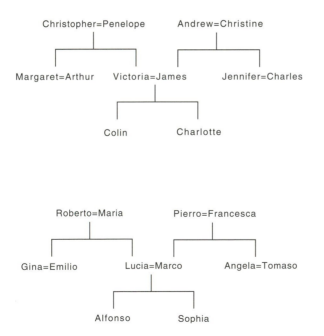

Figure 8.8   Two isomorphic family trees for an English and an Italian family that are used as a source of relationships for a feedforward network. (After Rumelhart et al., 1986; used with permission from *Nature*, copyright © 1986 Macmillan Magazines Ltd.)

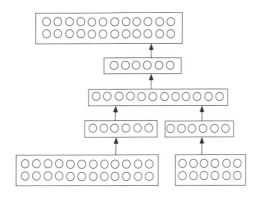

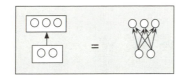

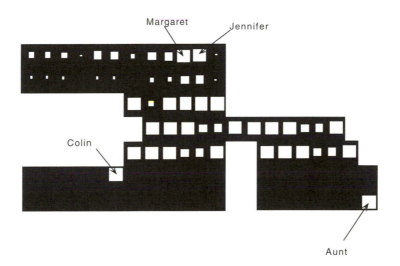

Figure 8.9 A four-layered network used to learn family trees. The legend shows the shorthand used to denote the connection patterns.

Figure 8.10 The activation pattern in the network after it has been trained. The input (*Colin, aunt*) is represented by turning on the appropriate units representing the person and the relationship. The output shows that the two units most activated represent Colin's aunts. The amount of activation is proportional to the size of the square. The units are arranged in the same pattern as they were in the previous figure. (After Rumelhart et al., 1986; used with permission from *Nature,* © 1986 Macmillan Magazines Ltd.)

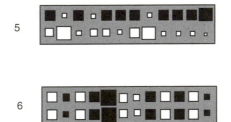

Figure 8.11 The weights for two hidden units in the second layer of the network that are connected to the input person units. The person units that the weights are from are shown in the key. The upper weights are from the English persons, as shown. The lower weights are from corresponding Italians. Positive weights are encoded as white squares and negative weights as black squares. The size of the square is proportional to the magnitude of the weight. (After Rumelhart et al., 1986; used with permission from *Nature,* © 1986 Macmillan Magazines Ltd.)

These are shown in Figure 8.11. As shown by the weight patterns, one of the units differentiates the country of the person, coding inputs from the English members with negative weights and inputs from the Italian members with positive weights. The weights from the other unit encode the left-hand side of the family trees. The point is that these units were not directly "told" to form these weight patterns. Instead, the fact that only a small number of units are used forces the network to encode the data. Consider that there are 288 possible input pairs but only 12 units at the center of the network. Thus the network units tend to respond to features that reflect underlying regularities in the data, such as nationality or a common lineage.

8.4 RECURRENT NETWORKS

The formulation for feedforward networks works owing to the unidirectional nature of the architecture. This allows the state variables to be a static function of the weights, and in turn allows the strategy of gradually adjusting the weights to be successful. But now suppose the networks have recurrent connections, as shown in Figure 8.12. Here the state variables are changing as the activation is propagated through the network. Can backpropagation still be used? It turns out that the trick of

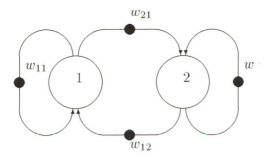

Figure 8.12 A very simple recurrent network with two units and four weights. (From Simard, 1991.)

translating time into space can still be used here, but now for each node in the network.[5]

The formulation of the equations will be analogous to the static case, the only difference being that, because the network is unrolled in time, the different levels correspond to different times. Consequently, the value of the weight for each unit must be the same regardless of the time step in which it appears.

To start, pick the following continuous activation equation:

$$T\frac{\partial x}{\partial t} = -x(t) + g[Wx(t)] + I(t)$$

In this equation T is a matrix of zeros with nonzero time constants on the diagonal; that is,

$$T = \begin{bmatrix} \tau_{11} & 0 & \cdots \\ 0 & \ddots & \\ \vdots & & \tau_{nn} \end{bmatrix}$$

The first step toward handling this equation is to discretize it. This is done by approximating the partial derivative as

$$\frac{\partial x}{\partial t} \approx \frac{x^{t+1} - x^t}{\Delta t}$$

where the different values of x are measured every Δt, so that the notation x^t means $x(t\Delta t)$. Thus the discretized equation is

$$x^{t+1} = x^t + \Delta t T^{-1}[-x^t + g(Wx^t) + I^t] \qquad (8.6)$$

This equation is the basis for understanding how a recurrent network can be transformed into a feedforward network. To see the relation more clearly, consider the network of Figure 8.12. This can be "unrolled" to produce the feedforward network shown by Figure 8.13, where time now translates into levels. In this network only the two units marked with the activation function g are nonlinear units. All the rest are linear. This example is of very modest size, but the point is that this strategy can be

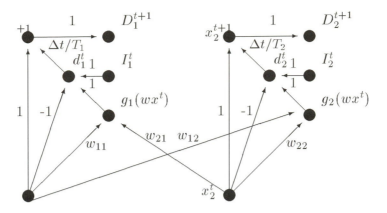

Figure 8.13 The feedforward model for the network in Figure 8.12. Shown is just one time step from t to $t + 1$. The corresponding "unrolled" model uses six units for each unit in the recurrent network. (From Simard, 1991.)

systematically applied to networks of arbitrary size. You should satisfy yourself that the figure is equivalent to Equation 8.6.

The development of the learning algorithm begins with the cost function. Pick the standard error function that measures the distance between the desired values and the actual values.

$$J = \frac{1}{2} \sum_{t=1}^{M} (S^t x^t - d^t)^T (S^t x^t - d^t)$$

Another difference from the static case is that the desired values might not all be defined at the final time but may be specified at arbitrary intermediate times.

The next step, which by now should appear very familiar, is to form the Hamiltonian. To do so, adjoin the dynamic equations to the cost function with Lagrange multipliers. Note that there are M such multipliers and that they must be vectors, as the state equation is in vector form.

$$H = J + \sum_{t=0}^{M-1} (\lambda^{t+1})^T \{ -x^{t+1} + x^t + \Delta t T^{-1} [-x^t + g(Wx^t) + I^t] \}$$

Now the next step is to find the adjoint equation

$$\left(\frac{\partial H}{\partial x^t} \right)^T = 0$$

$$= \begin{cases} S^t x^t - d^t - \lambda^t + (I - \Delta t T^{-1}) \lambda^{t+1} + \Delta t T^{-1} W^T \Lambda^{t+1} g'(Wx) \\ \quad \text{for } t = 0, \ldots, M - 1 \\ S^t x^M - d^M - \lambda^M \\ \quad \text{for } t = M \end{cases}$$

which, as usual, is solved backward in time. In this case,

$$\lambda^M = S^t x^M - d^M \tag{8.7}$$

$$\lambda^t = S^t x^t - d^t + (I - \Delta t T^{-1})\lambda^{t+1} + \Delta t T^{-1} W^T \Lambda^{t+1} g'(Wx) \tag{8.8}$$

$$\text{for } t = 0,\ldots, M - 1$$

The final step is to find the gradient of the Hamiltonian with respect to the weights. Some care is needed to navigate the very compact notation, but the result is

$$\left(\frac{\partial H}{\partial w_{ij}^t}\right)^T = \Delta t T^{-1} \sum_{t=0}^{M-1} \lambda_i^{t+1} x_j^t g_i'(w_i \cdot x^t) \tag{8.9}$$

As in the static case, solve the system equations by fixing the weights and propagating the solution through the network levels. Then solve the adjoint system for the λs going backward through the layers. Next adjust the weights according to their gradient. Continue until a convergence criterion is reached.

Example: A Recurrent Network for Learning XOR As a simple example consider the problem of learning the exclusive OR, or XOR, function shown in Table 8.2. This example is learned by a recurrent network with five units: two for the input, two hidden units, and one for the output. The signals are time-varying and defined for 25 time steps. The input units have a particular pattern applied continuously, and the output units are required to exhibit the correct response between time steps 10 and 15. Glance at the results of the network after training, shown in Figure 8.15, to get the idea. This shows the temporal trajectories. Note that they may wander around, but they hover near the correct values for the appropriate time steps.

Figure 8.14 shows the unrolled network for the first five time steps. The five main columns of units represent, from left to right, the input, hidden, and output units. The weights between the time steps are shared. Each unit is connected to all the others and has its own threshold. Thus there are $30 = 6 \times 5$ weights altogether. The learning rate used is 0.03. The weights are initialized to random values between ± 2.

Figure 8.15 shows the results after 400 learning epochs. The time constant used for learning is $\tau = 3$. You can see the effects of training clearly. The network approximates the answer during the time steps 11 through 15 but deviates owing to the unconstrained dynamics outside of this interval.

Table 8.2 Table for XOR.

$x_1 x_2$	y
0 0	0
0 1	1
1 0	1
1 1	0

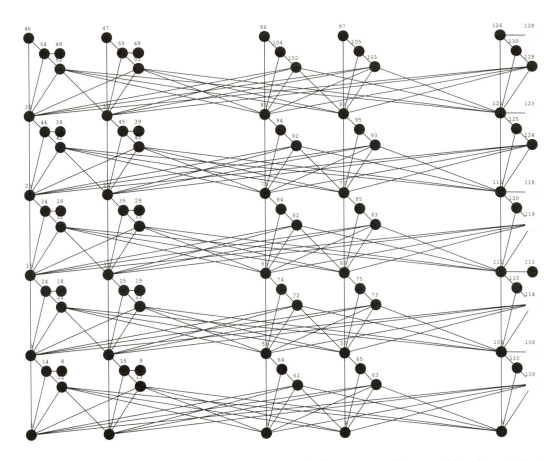

Figure 8.14 Unrolling the XOR network for five time steps. The network has five units that are arrayed horizontally. Time proceeds vertically. (From Simard, 1991.)

8.5 MINIMUM DESCRIPTION LENGTH

The notational complexity of feedforward and recurrent networks makes it easy to lose sight of the relationship between the Euler-Lagrange formulation and the ubiquitous minimum description length principle. The connections are as follows. One can think of the model output patterns as prototypes. The cost of the model is in terms of the network units and weights. If the model encodes the data exactly, the input pattern should produce the desired response. If it is close, the output can be thought of as a residual. The mathematical treatment in Section 2.6 covers precisely this case when the residual is normally distributed.

The number of units is prechosen by the designer, but they can be determined by mathematical principles based on eigenvalues.[6] As for the weights, there is an issue of precision. If the weights can have arbitrarily large precision, then the size of the model is unconstrained. One way to measure this cost is to add a penalty term to the objective function of the form $\|W\|$, which measures the bits in the weights. The form of such a function has been studied by Richard Zemel.[7]

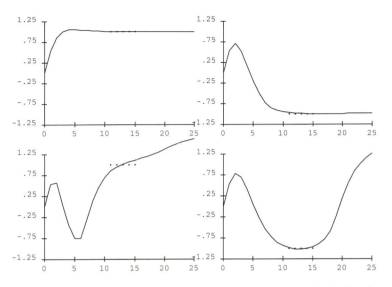

Figure 8.15 The results of learning XOR with recurrent networks. Reading from left to right and top to bottom, the four graphs show the recurrent network output unit's response to inputs that are (1, 1), (−1, 1), (−1, −1), and (1, −1), respectively, throughout the 25-step time period. The output unit's trajectory is constrained only for time steps 11 through 15, as shown by the dots. The dynamics of the system, together with the optimization function, allow the trajectories to wander when they are unconstrained. (From Simard, 1991.)

8.6 THE ACTIVATION FUNCTION

The motivation for introducing the sigmoidal activation function was that it was nonlinear and differentiable. But there are two other motivations for its form that will be discussed here. Both of these illustrate that for certain types of problems, the sigmoidal activation function simplifies the computation that has to be done. The setting is that of a two-layered network with sigmoidal activation function at the output layer.

8.6.1 Maximum Likelihood with Gaussian Errors

Suppose that there are two classes, y_1 and y_2. The network will have two output units, and we would like them to have activations that are equal to $P(y_1 \mid x)$ and $P(y_2 \mid x)$, respectively.[8] Recall that, from Bayes' rule

$$P(y_1 \mid x) = \frac{P(x \mid y_1)P(y_1)}{P(x)}$$

which can be written as

$$P(y_1 \mid x) = \frac{P(x \mid y_1)P(y_1)}{P(x \mid y_1)P(y_1) + P(x \mid y_2)P(y_2)}$$

$$= \frac{1}{1 + \frac{P(x \mid y_2)P(y_2)}{P(x \mid y_1)P(y_1)}}$$

Now introduce the exponential function, so that

$$P(y_1 \mid x) = \frac{1}{1 + e^{-\log\left[\frac{P(x|y_1)P(y_1)}{P(x|y_2)P(y_2)}\right]}} \tag{8.10}$$

This is already close to the answer we are looking for, as the right-hand side has the form of the sigmoid function $f(u) = \frac{1}{1 + e^{-u}}$, but there is a further simplification when the underlying distributions are Gaussian. Consider that these distributions are both characterized by

$$P(x \mid y_i) = \frac{1}{(2\pi)^{-\frac{n}{2}}|\Sigma|^{\frac{1}{2}}} e^{-\frac{1}{2}(x-m_i)^T \Sigma^{-1}(x-m_i)}$$

Substituting this equation into Equation 8.10 results in

$$P(y_1 \mid x) = \frac{1}{1 + e^{-w^T x + c}} \tag{8.11}$$

where

$$w = \Sigma^{-1}(m_1 - m_2)$$

and

$$c = \frac{1}{2}(m_1 - m_2)^T \Sigma^{-1}(m_1 - m_2) + \log \frac{P(y_1)}{P(y_2)}$$

So, for the rather special case of two Gaussian distributions with equal covariance matrices, the sigmoidal output units combine the input in just the right way. Given the means, covariance matrix, and *a priori* class probabilities, the network weights can be chosen so that the output activation is $P(y_i \mid x)$.

8.6.2 Error Functions

The second interesting case of the use of sigmoid functions occurs when the goal is to classify patterns into binary output vectors. Suppose that the desired output vector is d and the actual output vector is y. Then given the input x, the probability $P(d \mid x)$ can be written as

$$P(d \mid x) = \prod_i y_i^{d_i}(1 - y_i)^{1-d_i}$$

According to the Bayesian version of the MDL principle, the right thing to do is to minimize $-\log P$; in other words,

$$E = -\Sigma_i d_i \log y_i + (1 - d_i) \log (1 - y_i)$$

Taking the derivative of E with respect to the input of the unit u results in

$$\frac{\partial E}{\partial u} = \frac{d_i - y_i}{y_i(1 - y_i)} \frac{\partial f}{\partial u}$$

where $y_i = f(u_i)$ is assumed to be the activation function. Now, since for sigmoidal activation functions $\frac{\partial f}{\partial u_i} = y_i(1 - y_i)$,

$$\frac{\partial E}{\partial u} = d_i - y_i$$

Thus for the special case of binomially distributed errors, and changing the gradient according to the MDL error function (ignoring model costs), the gradient of the activation fortuitously cancels terms in the denominator so that the gradient of the error function is just linearly proportional to the difference between the desired output and the actual output.

NOTES

1. The perceptron was the brainchild of Frank Rosenblatt and was introduced in his book *Principles of Neurodynamics: Perceptrons and the Theory of Brain Mechanisms* (Washington, DC: Spartan Books, 1962). Marvin Lee Minsky and Seymour Papert demonstrated its limitations in *Perceptrons: An Introduction to Computational Geometry* (Cambridge, MA: MIT Press, 1969).

2. In the general form you want some margin, say $N\kappa$ (a constant κ is scaled by the number of components of the pattern). This is enforced by requiring that

$$w \cdot z^p > N\kappa$$

Thus the *perceptron learning rule* is given by

$$\Delta w = \mu\Theta[N\kappa - w \cdot z^p]z^p$$

3. The backpropagation algorithm has had a lively recent history. It was independently discovered by Werbos and Parker, but its importance with respect to the problem of multilayered networks was not appreciated until Rumelhart, Hinton, and Williams. More recently, Le Cun and Simard have shown its relation to classical control theory. P. Werbos, "Beyond Regression: New Tools for Prediction and Analysis in the Behavioral Sciences," Ph.D. thesis, Harvard University, 1974; D. Parker, "Learning Logic," TR 47, Center for Computational Research in Economics and Management Science, Massachusetts Institute of Technology, 1985; D. E. Rumelhart, G. E. Hinton, and R. J. Williams, "Learning Representations by Back-Propagating Errors," *Nature* 323 (1986):533–36; Y. Le Cun, "Une Procédure d'Apprentissage pour Réseau à Seuil Assymétrique," *Cognitiva 85: A la Frontiére de l'Intelligence Artificielle des Sciences de la Connaissance des Neurosciences*, pp. 599–604 (Paris, CESTA, 1985); Patrice Y. Simard, "Learning State Space Dynamics in Recurrent Networks," TR 383 and Ph.D. thesis, Computer Science Department, University of Rochester, 1991.

4. Rumelhart, Hinton, and Williams, "Learning Representations by Back-Propagating Errors."

5. The exposition of recurrent networks here was first developed by Patrice Simard in his doctoral dissertation, "Learning State Space Dynamics in Recurrent Networks."

6. Yann Le Cun, John S. Denker, and Sara A. Solla, "Optimal Brain Damage," in David S. Touretzky, ed., *Advances in Neural Information Processing Systems*, vol. 2 (San Mateo, CA: Morgan Kaufmann, 1990, pp. 598–605).

7. Richard S. Zemel, "A Minimum Description Length Framework for Unsupervised Learning," Ph.D. thesis, Computer Science Department, University of Toronto, 1993.

8. After M. I. Jordan, "Why the Logistic Function? A Tutorial Discussion on Probabilities and Neural Networks," Computational Cognitive Science Technical Report 9503, Massachusetts Institute of Technology, August 1995.

EXERCISES

1. Show graphically that AND is linearly separable, but that XOR is not where

$x_1 x_2$	y
0 0	0
0 1	0
1 0	0
1 1	1

2. In the simplest version of the perceptron learning rule, we want $w \cdot z^p > 0$ to hold for each pattern p. If it does not, we change w by an amount $\Delta w = -\eta (w \cdot z^p) z^p$ where $w \cdot z^p = w_1 z_1^p + w_2 z_2^p$. How large should η be to just correct the misclassification of the pattern shown in Figure 8.16 in one step?

3. For

$$g(u) = \frac{1}{1 + e^{-u}}$$

verify that

$$\frac{dg}{du} = g(u)[1 - g(u)]$$

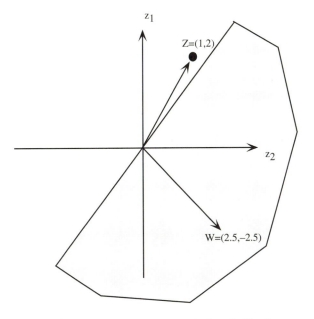

Figure 8.16 A particular situation to be handled by the perceptron learning rule.

4. Suppose, in the backpropagation algorithm, that the classes of the patterns are the outputs. Further suppose that it is desirable to maximize between-class separation and minimize within-class separation. Derive the appropriate error propagation formulae.

5. Verify the correctness of Equations 8.7 through 8.9 by expanding the vector equations into their scalar form.

6. Given the equation for recurrent networks,

$$H = J + \sum_{t=0}^{M-1} (\lambda^{t+1})^T \{ -x^{t+1} + x^t + \Delta t T^{-1}[-x^t + g(Wx^t) + I^t] \}$$

suppose that the time constants represented in the matrix T are also free parameters. Show how to modify them using gradient descent by differentiating the above equation with respect to τ_i.

7. Linearize the equation

$$T \frac{\partial x}{\partial t} = -x(t) + g[Wx(t)] + I(t)$$

about the point x_o and show for what values of T it is stable.

8. Show that with linear activation functions, a multilayered network is equivalent to a single-layered network.

9. Add a term that measures the cost of the weights, for example,

$$\sum_{i=1}^{n} \sum_{j=1}^{n} \sum_{k=1}^{K} (w_{ij}^k)^2$$

to the objective function and show how the equations used by Algorithm 8.1 are changed.

10. In many applications of networks, the input pattern is in the form of an image. In such cases it is desirable that the network recognize patterns, even when they have undergone small transformations. One way to incorporate this constraint into the networks is to add a term to the error function that measures the effect of the transformations explicitly (from Patrice Simard, Bernard Victorri, Yann Le Cun and John S. Denker, "Tangent Prop—A Formalism for Specifying Selected Invariances in an Adaptive Network," in John E. Moody, Steve J. Hanson, and Richard P. Lippmann, eds., *Advances in Neural Information Processing Systems*, vol. 4 [San Mateo, CA: Morgan Kaufmann, 1992, pp. 895–903]). That is, given pattern x, let $s(x, a)$ be the pattern rotated by a. Then you can add an error term to the standard error term that is weighted by a factor μ, that is

$$\mu \frac{\partial s}{\partial a}$$

Describe how you could compute this derivative and also how you could incorporate its effects into Algorithm 8.1.

11. If there are too many hidden units in a network, it may not generalize as well as it could, because the units tend to memorize individual patterns instead of capturing features between patterns. One way to force better generalization is to drop the weights (synapses) that are contributing the least (from Yann Le Cun, John S. Denker and Sara A. Solla, "Optimal Brain Damage," in David S. Touretzky, ed., *Advances in Neural Information Processing Systems*, vol. 2 [San Mateo, CA: Morgan Kaufmann, 1990, pp. 598–605]). To do this in a systematic way would require computing the Hessian, but this is impractical for large networks. An approximation to the Hessian involves computing its diagonal terms, that is

$$\frac{\partial^2 H}{\partial w_{ij}^2}$$

If this can be done, then weights with small values of the Hessian approximation can be dropped. Where the input to a network is given by

$$x_i = g(u_i)$$

and

$$u_i = \sum_j w_{ij} x_j$$

show that

$$\frac{\partial^2 H}{\partial w_{ij}^2} = \frac{\partial^2 H}{\partial u_i} x_j^2$$

and that the second derivatives between two layers are related by

$$\frac{\partial^2 H}{\partial u_i} = g'(u_i)^2 \sum_k w_{ki}^2 \frac{\partial^2 H}{\partial u_k^2} - g''(u_i) \frac{\partial H}{\partial x_i}$$

At the last layer, show that this becomes

$$\frac{\partial^2 H}{\partial u_i} = 2g'(u_i)^2 - 2(d_i - x_i)g''(u_i)$$

9 Unsupervised Learning

ABSTRACT In *unsupervised* learning, the only source of information is redundancy in the input signal. This redundancy can be exploited to encode the data efficiently. One way is to find *principal components*. A second way is by the use of a *classifier* that uses topological neighbors and multimodal data. A third way is to compute *independent components*.

9.1 INTRODUCTION

The previous chapter showed how heteroassociative memories with generalization capabilities could be learned if a set of known pairings could be used as a training set of data. However, in most biological settings, the pairings are not known but must be inferred from unlabeled data samples. In this *unsupervised* case the only source of information is redundancy in the input signal. This redundancy can be used to build compact representations. The principal ways of doing this were introduced in Chapter 4. Here these methods are implemented and extended in terms of networks.

We first show that a simple network can extract principal components from the data. This method allows the selection of a natural coordinate system in terms of the eigenvectors of the covariance matrix. Principal components is a "global" method in that all the components are used to encode a data point.

The global structure of principal components can make it difficult to recognize the difference between similar situations that require different responses. For that purpose the local structure of a classifier is useful. Prototype points provide a natural geometry for classifying data in that the input data are placed in the class of the nearest prototype.

A set of prototype points in the plane can be separated by line segments that bisect the lines joining closest points, as shown in Figure 9.1. The collection of all such segments is known as a *Voronoi diagram*. The collection of segments that join the prototype points and cross the bisectors is known as the *Delaunay triangulation* of the plane and in general as the dual of the Voronoi diagram. Given this structure, for any data point, the classification of the nearest prototype point (or k-nearest prototype points) can be selected as the class for that point. The Voronoi diagram shows the regions for which each prototype point is the closest and thus is similar to the basin of attraction introduced in Chapter 8.

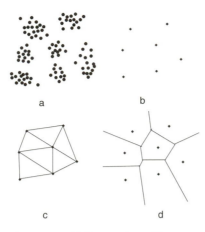

Figure 9.1 (*a*) Data points; (*b*) prototype points; (*c*) Delaunay triangulation; (*d*) Voronoi diagram.

Competitive learning is a general way to place prototypical points in noisy data. In this basic learning strategy, prototypes compete to represent the sensory patterns. This competition can be greatly improved if information is shared among topological neighbors. This is the basis of *Kohonen learning*.

Up to this point in the discussion, the model of the data is of a single real-valued state vector. However, a natural biological condition is that of *multimodal cues*. In this case data come in terms of tuples of points that are temporally coincident. Learning using this representation can be done without supervision, yet achieves comparable performance to supervised algorithms.

The classifier assumes that the input is predominantly one class exemplar. However, in a more complex situation, the input may be regarded as the superposition of multiple simultaneous "causes." *Independent components* is a "local" method that models this case using higher-order statistics of the data.

9.2 PRINCIPAL COMPONENTS

Chapter 4 showed that maximizing the variance of data samples leads to the choice of coordinate frame aligned with the eigenvectors of the covariance matrix of the samples. However, to compute those vectors using the methods of that chapter requires inverting a matrix. If only a relatively small number of eigenvalues are required, the trick of reducing the dimensionality of the space developed in Section 4.6 can be used. However, for high-dimensional spaces, inverting a matrix is an unwelcome prospect.

It turns out that the eigenvectors and their associated eigenvalues can be computed using a two-layer neural network, such as is shown in Figure 9.2, and applying the data as input to the network incrementally.

The principal components network uses linear units; that is, units with an output y given by

$$y = \sum_{j=1}^{N} w_j x_j$$

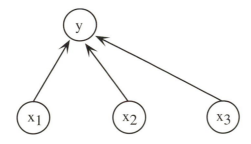

Figure 9.2 Two-layered network used to extract principal components.

For the moment, consider just one such unit. Starting from a given learning rule, we show that it almost does the right thing, and then provide the fix to make it find eigenvectors. The learning rule is the *Hebbian*[1] learning rule:

$$\Delta w_j = \eta y x_j \tag{9.1}$$

where η is a parameter that controls the learning rate. The way that this weight change is carried out is that the different samples x_j are applied in turn, and the adjustments to the weights are made sequentially. You will recognize this as just another application of the stochastic descent technique discussed in Chapter 8: Instead of pooling all the adjustments for each pattern, they are made in order, the hope being that this approach approximates pooling sufficiently well.

The effects of these adjustments can be seen by approximating Equation 9.1 with a continuous version that takes into account the effects of averaging over the different inputs x. For one pattern the approximation is

$$\dot{w}_j = \eta y x_j$$

Substituting for y,

$$= \eta \sum_{i=1}^{N} w_i x_i x_j$$

Now, averaging in the other samples,

$$\dot{w}_j = \eta \sum_{i=1}^{N} \sum_{k=1}^{M} w_i x_i^k x_j^k$$

or, considering all the components,

$$\dot{w} = \eta C w \tag{9.2}$$

where C is the correlation matrix. (If the patterns x_j had zero mean, C would be a covariance matrix.)

Since C is symmetric and positive semidefinite, all of its eigenvalues are positive or zero. Thus the solution to Equation 9.2 is unstable. Furthermore, the vector w will gradually line up with the eigenvector that has the largest eigenvalue. The direction of the eigenvector is the desired result except that its magnitude vector should be bounded instead of unbounded, as it is in the unstable system. One way to fix this problem would be to add a constraint on the length of w that is enforced during the optimization process. But there is a better way.[2]

The magnitude of the vector w can be constrained by modifying Equation 9.1 slightly to add a penalty term that discourages long vectors. The new rule becomes

$$\Delta w_j = \eta y(x_j - yw_j) \qquad (9.3)$$

It turns out that the algorithm implicitly defined by Equation 9.3 has several nice properties:

1. It converges to a weight vector of unit length, that is, $\|w\| = 1$.

2. The weight vector lies in the direction of the maximal eigenvector of C.

3. The weight vector lies in a direction that maximizes the variance of the data.

The algorithm given by Equation 9.3 finds just the largest eigenvalue and associated eigenvector, but it turns out that an elegant extension[3] can find the best k eigenvalues in descending order. Suppose there are k output units, one for each of k eigenvalues. Then the update rule becomes

$$\Delta w_{ij} = \eta y_i \left(x_j - \sum_{k=1}^{i} y_k w_{kj} \right) \qquad (9.4)$$

An Example: Representing Visual Images   As a concrete example of this technique, consider representing 8×8 pixel images by eigenfunctions. Such images can be obtained by taking random 8×8 patches from larger images. Each patch then represents a 64-element vector that serves as a training input x to a principal components network. The values of an output unit, after convergence of the algorithm, represent an eigenvalue of the covariance of the input samples. The corresponding weight vector represents the associated eigenvector. The eigenvectors are shown in Figure 9.3.[4]

9.3   COMPETITIVE LEARNING

The architecture of competitive learning is usually the same two-layered network that was used to extract principal components. The units labeled x_j represent the input space and a particular pattern in the input space is represented by the activation of those units and is denoted x. However, the weight update strategy is very different. The prototypes are labeled w_i. For any input pattern x, the unit that is closest to the input—that is, that w_i for which $\|w_i - x\|$ is minimum—is chosen as the prototype.

The number of units w_i is important, as that is the number of prototypes. The location of those prototypes, together with the distance metric, divides the space up into Voronoi regions, as shown in Figure 9.1. The prototype within each region is the closest for all the points in the region.

Competitive learning works incrementally. Given an input pattern, compute the closest prototype and then move the prototype closer to the

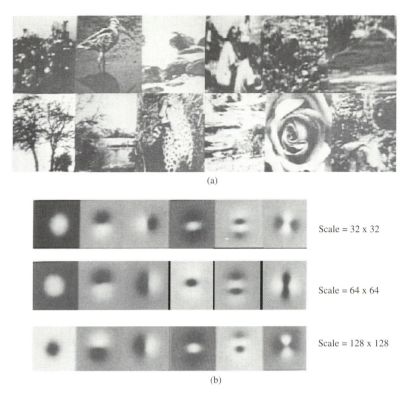

(a)

Scale = 32 x 32

Scale = 64 x 64

Scale = 128 x 128

(b)

Figure 9.3 Principal components for natural images found by using Equation 9.3. (From Hancock et al., 1992; used with permission of IOP Publishing Ltd.)

pattern. The "moving" is done by adjusting the weight from the input to the prototype so that the prototype responds more readily to that pattern. One can think of the prototype as being "captured" by a clump of patterns, where the net correction of all the patterns in the clump is zero. This process can be made more graphic by making the weights and input patterns directly comparable. They may be made comparable by normalizing both of them or, equivalently, projecting them onto the units sphere. In this case the prototype appears as a point in the same space as the patterns. Imagining that this procedure has been carried out, Figure 9.4 shows the effect of the data on a prototype as represented by its weights.

Formally this technique is described by Algorithm 9.1. In this algorithm, η is a learning rate that determines how far the prototype moves at each step.

Algorithm 9.1 Competitive Learning

For each pattern x,

1. Compute the closest prototype as the i that minimizes $\| w_i - x \|$.

2. Update the weight for that unit according to

$$\Delta w_i = \eta(x - w_i)$$

until Δw_i is sufficiently small.

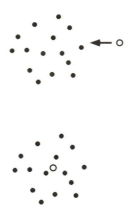

Figure 9.4 In competitive learning, data points compete for prototypes. Here a cluster of points attracts a prototype by producing a common correction for the prototype's weight vector.

The competitive learning algorithm can be thought of as a first try at solving the problem. It does fairly well, but it has two main problems:

1. There may be units that never win the competition. These occur as the weights have to be initialized with some strategy—randomizing them is one—and the chosen strategy may result in permanent losers.

2. The competitive learning algorithm is limited to a center-of-gravity strategy, positioning the prototypes in the middle of clumps of data. In simple cases this strategy could suffice, but for more complicated cases, where the patterns of data have complicated shapes that may interpenetrate, one would ideally like to have several prototypes per clump and position them near clump boundaries.

The intent of subsequent sections will be tackle these problems in order, each time improving the algorithm's performance.

9.4 TOPOLOGICAL CONSTRAINTS

The competitive learning algorithm treats all the prototype points as independent, but actually they have a natural topology in that some points are nearer to others. These relations can be used to make the learning algorithm both better and more efficient. The resultant algorithm is named after its discoverer, Teuvo Kohonen.

Kohonen learning solves the first problem of competitive learning, that of "dead" units. These are units that are never winners in the competitive scheme, and thus never have their weights adjusted. It solves this problem by adding the additional constraint of a topological neighborhood. In this case each of the prototype units has a set of neighbors. The winner moves toward the pattern, but so do the neighbors, albeit to a smaller extent. In this case all the units' receptive fields are adusted to be in the signal space and thus have a chance of being in the competition.

It would be a mistake to think of the Kohonen algorithm as just solving the problem of dead units. Under certain circumstances the topology itself can be the answer to a problem. Let us illustrate this principle with a specific example, the traveling salesman problem.

9.4.1 The Traveling Salesman Example

Given a set of cities $\{x_1, x_2\}$, the problem is to find a minimal-length tour that traverses all the cities, returning to the city of origin.

The way this is solved is shown in Algorithm 9.2, which uses a set of protoypes that are notionally connected on a ring. In other words, the prototypes define a tour. Initially this tour of prototypical cities is just placed at the center of the map, as shown in Figure 9.5, and does not correspond to any of the "data" cities. But as the computation proceeds, the prototype cities on the tour are pulled toward the input cities until finally they are in correspondence. When this condition is achieved, the computation ends and the cities on the ring can be read out in sequential order by proceeding along the ring.

Algorithm 9.2 Kohonen Learning Algorithm

Set α to a large number. While $\alpha \geq .001$, for each input city (x_1, x_2), do the following:

1. Find the nearest prototype city y_1, y_2.

2. If the nearest is unique, move it and its neighbors by

$$\Delta y_i = e^{-d^2/a}(y_i - x_i), i = 1, 2$$

otherwise, resolve the tie by duplicating a prototype city and allowing just one of the prototypes to move.

3. Decrease α.

In the formula for moving the prototype given in Algorithm 9.2, d is defined on the ring as the distance from the winner to the prototype city in question. The distance from the winner to itself is of course 0, the distance to the winner's two nearest neighbors is 1, the distance to their neighbors is 2, and so on. When a prototype city is between two data cities and is pulled in two different directions, the conflict is resolved by duplicating the prototype city. Then one copy of the original prototype moves toward one of the data cities, and the other copy moves toward that city's competitor.

9.4.2 Natural Topologies

In the traveling salesman problem, the definition of neighbors or *topology* of the internal units is determined by the requirements of the problem. Since the answer is to be a tour, a tour is encoded into the algorithm in

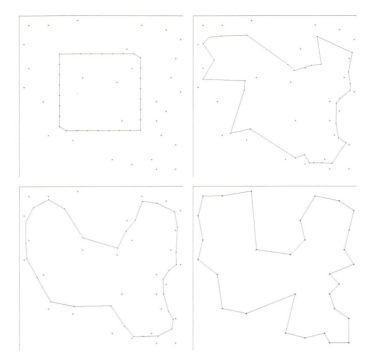

Figure 9.5 The Kohonen algorithm applied to the traveling salesman problem. Successive panels from left to right and top to bottom show stages in the convergence of the algorithm. (Courtesy of Robert Wisniewski.)

terms of predetermined and evolving neighborhood relationships. The more general case is that there is no natural neighborhood function that can be determined *a priori* but rather that the appropriate neighborhood function is defined in terms of the data themselves. Figure 9.6 shows an artificial example to illustrate this point. The figure shows an artificial distribution of input samples that can be three-dimensional, two-dimensional, or one-dimensional, depending on what part of the input space is being sampled. Thus the natural topology linking the samples that should represent the input distribution is space-variant.

The information needed to learn the desired topology is inherent in the input samples. For example, given the prototypes, a simple algorithm for finding it would be to find the nearest two prototypes for every sample and add that neighborhood relation to the set. This idea can be improved in two ways: (1) it can be extended to work with the discovery of the correct placement of prototypes by Kohonen learning; and (2) it can be made to work incrementally as each sample is considered. Thus neighborhood relations can be discovered based on the ongoing observed correlations.[5] This principle is the basis of Algorithm 9.3, which makes use of a connectivity matrix C. In this matrix $C_{ij} > 0$ if i and j are neighbors; otherwise $C_{ij} = 0$. Associated with each link ij is an age, stored in t_{ij}, that keeps track of the recency of the neighborhood estimate.

Chapter 9   Unsupervised Learning

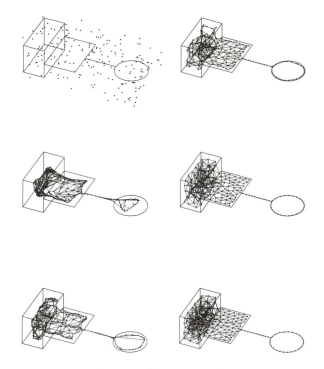

Figure 9.6 Performance of the topology discovery algorithm on an artificial input space with three-, two-, and one-dimensional correlation neighborhoods. (Reprinted from Martinetz and Schulten, 1994, *Neural Networks*, © 1994, with kind permission from Elsevier Science, Ltd., The Boulevard, Langford Lane, Kidlington, 0X5 1GB, UK.)

Algorithm 9.3 Competitive Topology Learning

Initialize the prototypes w_i, $i = 1,\dots,M$.

Initialize the connectivity matrix C_{ij} of connection strengths to 0.

For each input pattern x^μ and for each w_i, do the following:

1. Estimate k_i, the number of prototypes closer to x^μ than w_i, and find the two closest, w_{i0} and w_{i1}.

2. Update the weight for those units according to

$$\Delta w_{ij} = \eta e^{-k_i/\lambda}(x^\mu - w_{ij})$$

3. Update the connectivity information

a. set $C_{i_0 i_1} = 1$ and $t_{i_0 i_1} = 0$.

b. for all i and j such that $C_{ij} = 1$ increment t_{ij}.

c. for all j such that $C_{i_0 j} = 1$ and $t_{i_0 j} > T$ set $C_{i_0 j} = 0$.

until Δw_{i0} is sufficiently small.

The results of running the algorithm on test data are shown as an overlay in Figure 9.6. For this simulation, the parameter λ, the step size η, and

Table 9.1 Parameters used in topology-finding algorithm.

Parameter	Initial Value	Final Value
η	0.3	0.05
λ	$0.2N$	0.01
T	$0.1N$	$2N$

the lifetime T were time-dependent. The functional form of this dependence is the same for all parameters; for example, for η, it was

$$\eta(t) = \eta_i \left(\frac{\eta_f}{\eta_i} \right)^{t/t_{max}}$$

The number of prototype points used was 200. The parameter values used in the simulation appear in Table 9.1.

9.5 SUPERVISED COMPETITIVE LEARNING

We can now tackle the more important of the two problems with competitive learning, namely, that the placement of the prototype vectors cannot be guaranteed to be optimal with respect to a given task. In order to make headway, assume that the classes of the prototype vectors are known. In other words, the formulation is now supervised. In the unsupervised algorithm, prototypes were forced to move toward clumps of data. Supervision allows them to have more freedom of movement. Figure 9.7 shows a case where the natural clumps of data produced by the unsupervised learning algorithm are incorrect. It also shows that

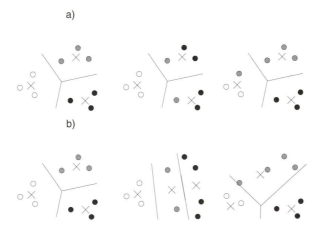

Figure 9.7 Unsupervised versus supervised learning. (*a*) Unsupervised competitive learning performs well when the desired classes are obvious from the data clusters, but makes mistakes otherwise. (*b*) The mistakes are corrected with supervision. (From de Sa, 1994.)

the correct classification of data can be obtained if supervision is allowed.

If you think of the data from different classes as having two different probability distributions, the best thing to do would be to have the separation boundary be at a point between the two local distributions that minimizes some criterion. Given such a criterion, supervised algorithms adjust the separation boundary by sampling input near the current border and using the criterion to decide the best way to move it. As an aid to remembering that this algorithm is supervised, the prototype vectors are termed *codebook vectors*.

Let us choose the criterion of minimizing misclassifications. This criterion can be represented by the following objective function, which counts the number of errors:

$$E(b) = \int_b^\infty P(C_1)p(x \mid C_1)dx + \int_{-\infty}^b P(C_2)p(x \mid C_2)dx \qquad (9.5)$$

where $P(C_i)$ is the *a priori* probability of class i and $p(x \mid C_i)$ is the probability density function for x given class i. To explain the algorithm, it helps to think of moving the borders between codebook vectors, in this case b, rather than the vectors themselves.

Now to minimize $E(b)$, differentiate with respect to b:

$$\frac{dE}{db} = P(C_2)p(x \mid C_2) - P(C_1)p(x \mid C_1)$$

This cannot be solved for b, but the right b might be found by gradient descent. That is, you would incrementally adjust b by

$$\Delta b = -\eta \frac{dE}{db}$$

Now it is impractical to use this method also, but the idea is very close to the practical answer. It turns out that there is a simple procedure that approximates this gradient descent (although the proof that it works is involved). At every iteration change b by

$$\Delta b = \eta Z$$

where Z is given by

$$Z = \begin{cases} 1 & \text{if } x \in C_1 \text{ and } |x - b| < c \\ -1 & \text{if } x \in C_2 \text{ and } |x - b| < c \\ 0 & \text{otherwise} \end{cases}$$

Figure 9.8 shows the use of the algorithm for a hypothetical situation where a pattern near the border separating two clusters of points has been misclassified. The prototype points are moved in a direction that increases the chances of correctly classifying the point. These relations are used in Algorithm 9.4.

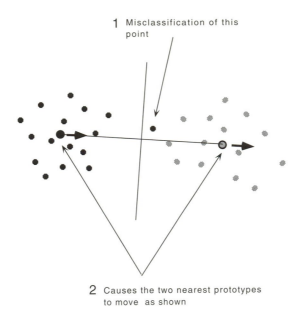

1 Misclassification of this
point

2 Causes the two nearest prototypes
to move as shown

Figure 9.8 The supervised competitive learning algorithm works by moving prototypes to improve classification performance.

Algorithm 9.4 Supervised Competitive Learning

For each input x find its two nearest codebook vectors, w_1 and w_2.

If they are from different classes and the input is near the border separating them, do the following:

1. Move the codebook vector from the correct class 1 toward the pattern; that is,

$$\Delta w_1 = \eta \frac{(x - w_1)}{\|x - w_1\|}$$

2. Move the incorrect class 2 away from the pattern; that is,

$$\Delta w_2 = -\eta \frac{(x - w_2)}{\|x - w_2\|}$$

9.6 MULTIMODAL DATA

Supervised competitive learning performs well, but there is still motivation to do without the class labels, especially since such labels are not always available. There is a way to do without the labels, but it only works if you are close to the right answer. Fortunately the same strategy also allows finding a good initial approximation. This strategy assumes that data come in sets of pairs or more. This is usually the case for biological situations, owing to the *multimodal* nature of stimuli. The sensations of sight, hearing, touch, and smell usually occur together. The development here will focus on just two modalities, but the extension to more than two is straightforward.

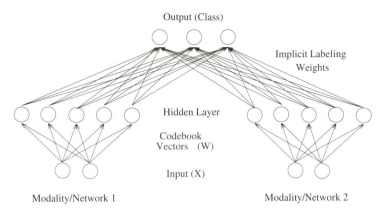

Figure 9.9 Multimodal architecture. (From de Sa, 1994.)

The multimodal constraint can be utilized by adding a layer to join two of the two-layered networks of the kind described by Figure 9.2. The resultant architecture is shown in Figure 9.9. This architecture can be used in two phases. First, the temporal coincidence between two inputs from different modalities can be used to assign initial class prototypes. As shown in Figure 9.7, the protoypes placed in this way are unlikely to be optimal. This is the motivation for the second phase. During this later phase, an objective function is used to place the prototypes at locations that are good for classifying new data.

9.6.1   Initial Labeling Algorithm

The prototypes can be selected using the competitive learning algorithm. A vector from each modality is applied to the two input networks, and two corresponding "class-prototype" vectors are selected. Each of these activates units at the top layer, and one of these is selected as the winner and has its weights updated. After a set of pairs has been applied to the network, an initial set of prototypes will have been chosen. The competitive learning algorithm needs to be applied to the last two layers of the network only, but this step is easy to do.

9.6.2   Minimizing Disagreement

Assuming that the prototypes are initially placed, the next step is to try to adjust their locations to optimize their usefulness in classifying new data.

Consider the simplest case of just pairs of stimuli, each of a single dimension, and two classes. This situation is shown in Figure 9.10. In this case, when modality 1 experiences a stimulus from pattern class A, then modality 2 will also experience a pattern from class A. Similarly, patterns from class B will co-occur in time for each of the two modalities. The situation is very similar to the supervised case, with the essential modification

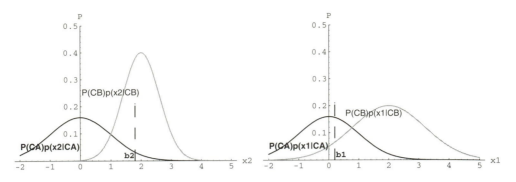

Figure 9.10 A simple case of multimodal pattern discrimination. (From de Sa, 1994.)

of now having the two sensory systems. Thus instead of one boundary to move, there are now two, one for each modality.[6]

In the supervised case, knowing the class labels allowed the use of an error metric that minimized the number of misclassified patterns. Knowing the classes was the key that allowed the use of this metric. In the multimodal case, since the goal is to derive an unsupervised algorithm, the class labels cannot be used, but there is a similar idea, termed *disagreement error:* the number of patterns classified differently by the two networks. The logic behind this idea is that the co-occurring patterns should be classified the same, so that any disagreements are naturally errors. Disagreement error can be written as follows:

$$E(b_1, b_2) = P\{x_1 < b_1 \ \& \ x_2 > b_2\} + P\{x_1 > b_1 \ \& \ x_2 < b_2\}$$

The easiest way to think about disagreement error is to work with the joint density function $f(x_1, x_2)$. This is defined as

$$f(x_1, x_2) = p(x_1 \mid C_A)p(x_2 \mid C_A)P(C_A) + p(x_1 \mid C_B)p(x_2 \mid C_B)P(C_B)$$

Now consider the domain of this function, together with the two boundaries b_1 and b_2. To compute the appropriate error measure, it suffices to integrate over the regions that represent disagreements in the classes. Formally,

$$E(b_1, b_2) = \int_{-\infty}^{b_1} \int_{b_2}^{\infty} f(x_1, x_2)dx_1 dx_2 + \int_{b_1}^{\infty} \int_{-\infty}^{b_2} f(x_1, x_2)dx_1 dx_2$$

Minimizing this function using gradient descent would require that the derivatives with respect to b_1 and b_2 be computed. These are

$$\frac{\partial E}{\partial b_1} = \int_{b_2}^{\infty} f(b_1, x_2)dx_2 - \int_{-\infty}^{b_2} f(b_1, x_2)dx_2$$

Similarly,

$$\frac{\partial E}{\partial b_2} = \int_{b_1}^{\infty} f(x_1, b_2)dx_1 - \int_{-\infty}^{b_1} f(x_1, b_2)dx_1$$

One way to perform gradient descent would be to use a lot of samples of x_2 to estimate $\frac{\partial E}{\partial b_1}$, and similarly for $\frac{\partial E}{\partial b_2}$. A better way, however, is to make an adjustment after each individual sample. The idea is that the sum of the adjustments is equivalent to the adjustment using the sum. Thus, as before, the borders can be moved by

$$\Delta b_1 = \eta Z \tag{9.6}$$

where z is given by

$$Z = \begin{cases} 1 & \text{if } X_2 < b_2 \text{ and } |x - b_1| < c \\ -1 & \text{if } X_2 > b_2 \text{ and } |x - b_1| < c \\ 0 & \text{otherwise} \end{cases} \tag{9.7}$$

These relations are used in Algorithm 9.5.

Algorithm 9.5   Unsupervised Competitive Learning

For each modality j do the following:

1. For each input X_j find its two nearest codebook vectors, w_{j1} and w_{j2}.

2. If they are from different classes and the input is near the border separating them, then move the codebook vectors as follows:

$$\Delta w_{1j} = \eta \frac{(X_1 - w_{1j})}{\|X_1 - w_{1j}\|}$$

$$\Delta w_{2j} = -\eta \frac{(X_1 - w_{2j})}{\|X_1 - w_{2j}\|}$$

Note that the only major change here is that the border b_2 is playing the role of the class information in counseling the movement of b_1. If modality 2 decides upon "class A" ($X_2 < b_2$), then the classifier for modality 1 increases its chance of saying "class A" by moving its border b_1 to the right. On the other hand, if the modality 2 classifier decides on "class B," then it decreases the chance of the modality 1 classifier saying "class A" by moving the border to the left. Naturally there are equations similar to Equations 9.6 and 9.7 for Δb_2 and its corresponding Z.

This development is for the one-dimensional case and uses two classes. What happens when the dimensionality is much larger and several classes are involved? It happens that the one-dimensional result can be used to approximate this situation. In the larger case, the individual data points activate the two nearest prototypes of different classes, and the algorithm is applied to adjust those two points. Figure 9.11 shows a hypothetical situation for two dimensions and two modalities. Note that points in this diagram occur in pairs, one for each modality. Corresponding prototypes can be given a common label by virtue of their participation in a competitive learning algorithm. Given a pattern, network 1 does not have a class label for that pattern, but can use the class label determined by network 2.

Similarly, network 2 does not have a class label for the corresponding input pattern, but can use the class label determined by network 1.

Example: Simultaneous Visual and Acoustic Signals   The multimodal algorithm is illustrated with the following experiment (carried out by its inventor, Virginia de Sa). Simultaneous visual and auditory signals were recorded from five male English speakers as they spoke the syllables /ba/, /va/, /da/, /ga/, and /wa/.

The images are digitized video signals that were then preprocessed to obtain 25 equally spaced samples that measure local image motion. Five frames of video were used to obtain a visual modality data vector of 125 samples. Examples of the /ba/ and /va/ utterances are shown in Figure 9.12.

The acoustic data were sampled for nine steps of 20-millisecond windows. The speech signal was encoded as a 24-channel mel code, resulting in a 216-dimension auditory data vector.

Figure 9.13 shows the results of several experiments. The results are plotted in groups of four, representing, from left to right, the results of the auditory training set, the auditory test set, the visual training set, and the visual test set. The leftmost two groups of four show the results of using just a single speaker. For this case 100 samples were used as a training set

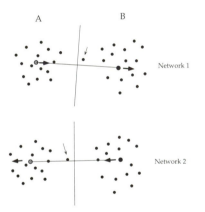

Figure 9.11   How the minimum-disagreement rule works. Network 1 uses the classification of network 2 (*A*) in deciding whether to shift its boundary by moving the prototypes. Similarly, network 2 uses the classification of network 1 (*B*) in its decision.

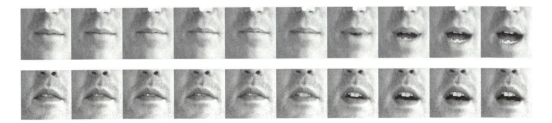

Figure 9.12   Examples of the utterances /ba/ and /va/. (From de Sa, 1994.)

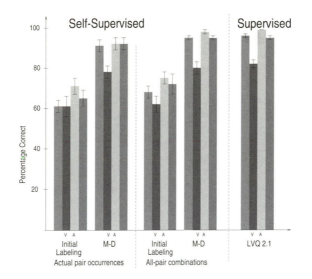

Figure 9.13 Results on the single-speaker cross-modal data set. The two leftmost bars in each set of four give the performance of the visual network, and the rightmost bars show the auditory network's performance. Within the two bars for each modality, the lighter, leftmost bars represent performance on the training set. The darker, rightmost bars give results on the test set. The error bars represent one standard deviation. (From de Sa, 1994.)

and an additional 20 as a test set. The leftmost set of four bars shows the result of just using temporal coincidence in a competitive learning algorithm. The adjacent set of four bars shows the improvement obtained by subsequently applying the minimum disagreement algorithm.

The next two sets of four show the results for combining all the pairs from a single speaker, even when they did not occur simultaneously. These provide an estimate of the possible improvement of the algorithm with additional data. For comparison, the results on the same data obtained with the supervised competitive algorithm are shown in the rightmost set of four bars.

9.7 INDEPENDENT COMPONENTS

In independent components analysis, the world is assumed to be composed of hidden but independent causes or *sources s*. These causes are experienced as data owing to the transform $x = As$. The columns of the matrix A are basis functions that specify how each cause weights a particular component of the data vector. Thus a compact code would be one that recovers the original causes.

If the perceptual system were linear, then the code could be represented in terms of units u such that

$$u = Wx$$

By direct substitution it is easy to see that

$$u = Wx = WAs$$

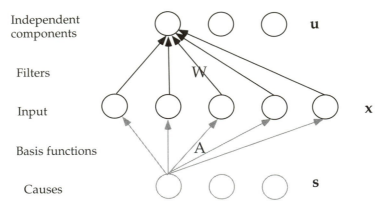

Independent components

Filters

Input

Basis functions

Causes

$\mathbf{u}$

W

$\mathbf{x}$

A

$\mathbf{s}$

Figure 9.14 The architecture behind the independent components. The world is assumed to be composed of hidden but independent causes s that are seen as data owing to the transform $x = As$. The job of independent components analysis is to factor the data into its independent causes such that $W = A^{-1}$.

so that if $W = A^{-1}$, then u would represent the sources. Thus the job of independent components analysis is to factor the data into its independent causes such that $W = A^{-1}$ (see Figure 9.14).

A step toward getting independent components would be to have W be a decorrelating matrix. Such a matrix results in the covariance matrix of u being diagonal; that is, $E(uu^T)$ has only nonzero terms on the diagonal.

Consider the special case where $E(uu^T) = I$. Then

$$E(uu^T) = I = E(Wxx^TW^T)$$

so that

$$W^TW = [E(xx^T)]^{-1} \tag{9.8}$$

Principal components can be seen as one such solution. In that solution,

$$\Phi\Lambda\Phi = E(xx^T) = \Sigma \tag{9.9}$$

Combining Equations 9.8 and 9.9,

$$W = \Lambda^{-\frac{1}{2}}\Phi^T$$

The principal components solution constitutes a code, but it does not take into account statistics above second-order or address the model of combined sources where the distribution of sources is given by

$$p(s) = \prod_{i=1}^{N} p_{s_i}(s_i)$$

A better criterion is to maximize the entropy $H(y)$ where y is a sigmoidally transformed version of x, that is, $y = g(x)$.[7] Now $p(y)$ can be written in terms of $p(x)$ by using the determinant of the Jacobian J:

$$p(y) = \frac{p(x)}{|J|} \tag{9.10}$$

where

$$J = \left| \frac{\partial y}{\partial x} \right|$$

Now since

$$H(y) = -E[\ln p(y)]$$

then using Equation 9.10,

$$H(y) = E[\ln |J|] + H(x)$$

Since x does not depend on the weights in the network, to minimize $H(y)$ one has to concentrate only on the first term on the right-hand side, so that a gradient ascent algorithm is given by

$$\Delta W = \eta \frac{\partial H(y)}{\partial W} = \eta E\left[\frac{\partial |J|}{\partial W} \right]$$

Once again you can use stochastic gradient ascent and calculate the gradient in an online manner. To perform this calculation, ignore the expectation operator in the preceding equation. This step results in[8]

$$\Delta W = \eta [(W^T)^{-1} + \hat{y}x^T]$$

In this formula $\hat{y}$ has elements

$$\hat{y}_i = \frac{\partial}{\partial y_i} \frac{\partial y_i}{\partial u_i}$$

where the activation function is the standard

$$y_i = \frac{1}{1 + e^{-u_i}}$$

Now, multiplying the gradient ascent equation by a matrix will just scale the gradient (albeit differently along the different dimensions). A matrix that is particularly useful is the symmetric matrix $W^T W$ because it gets rid of the inverse.[9] This derivation results in Algorithm 9.6.

Algorithm 9.6 Independent Components

Starting from a random initialization of the weights in a two-layered network, adjust the weights according to

$$\Delta W = \eta (I + \hat{y}x^T W^T) W$$

gradually decreasing the learning rate η.

NOTES

1. Donald O. Hebb pioneered the study of neural networks in the 1940s, in his book *The Organization of Behavior: A Neuropsychological Theory* (New York: Science Editions, 1949), laying out many of the basic criteria from which the formal developments recounted here have followed.

2. Found by E. Oja, in "Neural Networks, Principal Components, and Subspaces," *International Journal of Neural Systems* 1 (1989):61–68 and described in John Hertz, Anders Krogh, and Richard

G. Palmer, *Introduction to the Theory of Neural Computation*, Lecture Notes Volume 1, Santa Fe Institute Studies in the Sciences of Complexity (Redwood City, CA: Addison-Wesley, 1991).

3. Due to T. Sanger, "Optimal Unsupervised Learning in a Single-Layer Linear Feedforward Neural Network," *Neural Networks* 2 (1989):459–73.

4. Peter J. B. Hancock, Roland J. Baddeley, and Leslie S. Smith, "The Principal Components of Natural Images," *Network* 3 (1992):61–70.

5. This idea is due to Thomas Martinetz and Klaus Schulten, described in "Topology Representing Networks," *Neural Networks* 7, no. 3 (1994):507–22.

6. The disagreement minimization criterion is due to Virginia de Sa, and its presentation here is derived from the discussion in her thesis, "Unsupervised Classification Learning from Cross-Modal Environmental Structure," TR 536 and Ph.D. thesis, Computer Science Department, University of Rochester, November 1994.

7. For more details see Anthony J. Bell and Terrence J. Sejnowski, "Fast Blind Separation Based on Information Theory," *Proceedings of the 1995 International Symposium on Non-Linear Theory and Applications*, 1995, pp. 43–47.

8. Anthony J. Bell and Terrence J. Sejnowski, "An Information Maximization Approach to Blind Separation and Blind Deconvolution," *Neural Computation* 7 (1995):1129–59.

9. S. Amari, A. Cichocki, and H. H. Yang, "A New Learning Algorithm for Blind Signal Separation," in *Advances in Neural Information Processing Systems*, vol. 8 (Cambridge, MA: MIT Press, 1996).

EXERCISES

1. Test the principal components algorithm by using $N \times N$ samples from natural images as training data. Pick N appropriately for your computer. Plot the resultant receptive fields of the units w.

2. Show that for the principal components algorithm, variance maximization is equivalent to finding the maximal eigenvector.

3. Show that for the principal components algorithm given by Equation 9.3, the algorithm converges to an equilibrium value where $\|w\| = 1$ and λ is an eigenvalue of C.

4. Implement the traveling salesman problem using Kohonen learning and experimentally adjust the parameter α for best results.

5. State the conditions for a local minimum of $E(b_1, b_2)$ in multimodal unsupervised learning.

6. Show that for the sigmoid function used in the calculation of independent components,

$$\hat{y}_i = 1 - 2y$$

7. Test the independent components algorithm by mixing together two audio signals. That is, give a two-dimensional source s, and construct the input by using a mixing matrix A where

$$x(t) = As(t)$$

Next, use the algorithm to create an unmixed pair of signals $y(t)$.

III   Programs

Part III is about learning behavioral programs. Such learning necessarily requires longer timescales than do reactive memories that are dictated by short timescales. Given 50 milliseconds to work with, using devices that take on the order of 2–10 ms to send a voltage spike, there is little else to do but store computations in tables (synapses). One can think of these tables as representing primitive state-action pairs. However, given timescales of 300 ms to seconds, there are more options available. On this longer timescale one can begin to think of assembling sequences of such actions to form more complex behaviors.

Another reason for sequentiality is dictated by the structure of physical systems operating in space and time. An example is human eye movements. The human is forced to select a single gaze point out of a visual continuum. Examining an image necessitates sequential gaze points, thus saccades. That the brain does use such sequences is obvious from the study of eye movements.[1] Vision in humans involves continual sequential interactions with the world. The central characteristic of human vision is saccades. These are discrete eye movements made at the rate of about three per second. These movements can achieve speeds of about 700 degrees per second. Experiments have suggested that very little information is retained from image to image, and have shown that these movements are intimately related to subjects' momentary problem solving.[2] Thus at the 300-ms timescale cognition appears as sequential programs that depend on moment-by-moment interactions with the environment.

Sequentiality costs in time, but it can lead to enormously compact encodings, as an artificial example illustrates. Consider the task of determining the parity of an image of ones and zeros. Experiments show that the feedforward net requires a very large number of hidden units to determine parity, but a very small Turing machine can make this determination sequentially.

BRAIN SUBSYSTEMS THAT USE CHEMICAL REWARDS

We do not yet understand the details of how the brain coordinates sequential actions on the 300-ms timescale, yet so much new information about the various brain subsystems has recently been discovered that one can at least describe a broad picture of their functionality. Let us briefly describe the main ideas about key subsystems.

• The *basal ganglia* form an extensive subcortical nucleus implicated in the learning of motor program sequences. Neurons in the basal ganglia that respond to task-specific subsequences emerge in the course of training.[3] Most important, basal ganglia neurons learn to predict reward.[4] When a monkey initially reaches into an enclosed box for an apple, these neurons respond when the fingers touch the apple. If a light is paired with the apple reward in advance of reaching into the box, the same neurons develop responses to the light and not to the actual touching. These neurons are dopaminergic; that is, they are responsible for one of the main chemical reward systems used by the brain. Thus the implication is that the monkey is learning to predict delayed reward and coding it by means of an internal dopamine messenger. This secondary reward is used to signal the beginning of motor programs that lead to direct reward (Figure III.1).[5]

The basal ganglia have extensive connections to cortex that emphasize frontal and motor cortex (Figure III.2).[6]

• The *hippocampus* is an extensive subcortical nucleus implicated in the enabling of working memory. Lesions of the hippocampus allow the carrying out of tasks that require working memory but impair the ability to retain these memories.

The hippocampus has extensive connections to cortex that heavily emphasize abstract areas of cortex (Figure III.3).[7]

Broadly speaking, information about program sequence is represented in the basal ganglia,[8] and information as to the long-term retention of items in spatial working memory depends on the hippocampus.[9]

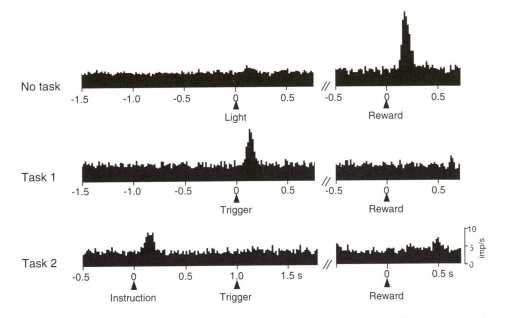

Figure III.1 Evidence of basal ganglia programming. A monkey is initially given a reward. At that time the secondary-reward neurons in the basal ganglia fire to record the reward event. Next the task is changed so that, at a start signal, the monkey must reach into a box for an apple. Now the same neuron hands out the secondary reward at the start of the task, rather than at the point of actual reward. Next the contingency is changed again, so that now a light indicates the presence or absence of reward in the box. Now the neuron hands out the secondary reward at the time of the positive cue. The inference is that the basal ganglia record the start of motor programs and that these are constantly being modified based on secondary-reward estimates. (From Schultz et al., 1995.)

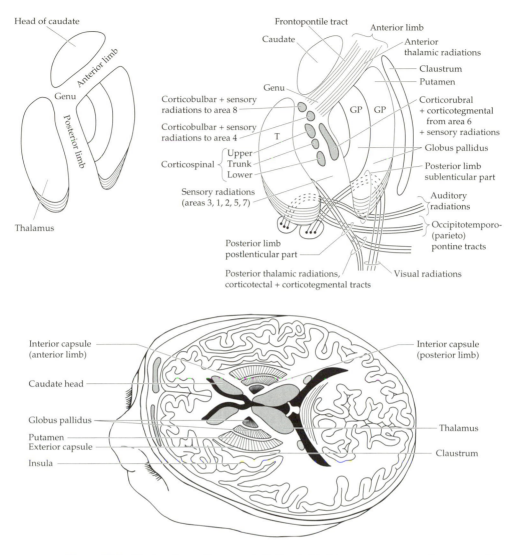

Head of caudate

Anterior limb

Genu

Posterior limb

Thalamus

Frontopontile tract

Caudate

Anterior limb

Anterior thalamic radiations

Genu

Claustrum

Putamen

Corticobulbar + sensory radiations to area 8

Corticobulbar + sensory radiations to area 4

Corticorubral + corticotegmental from area 6 + sensory radiations

Globus pallidus

GP GP

Corticospinal { Upper Trunk Lower

T

Posterior limb sublenticular part

Sensory radiations (areas 3, 1, 2, 5, 7)

Auditory radiations

Occipitotemporo-(parieto) pontine tracts

Posterior limb postlenticular part

Visual radiations

Posterior thalamic radiations, corticotectal + corticotegmental tracts

Interior capsule (anterior limb)

Interior capsule (posterior limb)

Caudate head

Globus pallidus

Thalamus

Putamen
Exterior capsule

Claustrum

Insula

Figure III.2 The basal ganglia are centrally located to interconnect motor subsystems with the cortex. (From Pansky and Allen, 1980; reproduced from *Review of Neuroscience*, © 1980 Macmillan, with permission of the McGraw-Hill Companies.)

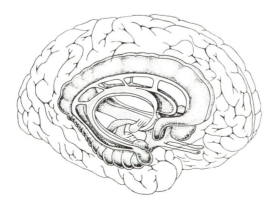

Figure III.3 The location and shape of the hippocampus, shown by the darkened area, facilitate interconnecting cortical areas. (From Pansky and Allen, 1980; reproduced from *Review of Neuroscience*, © 1980 Macmillan, with permission of the McGraw-Hill Companies.)

THE ROLE OF REWARDS

The operations seen in the basal ganglia are fundamental. In order to pre-dict the value of future rewards the brain must have an internal account-ing system that keeps track of the expected value of the current actions. As we have discussed, dopamine is one of the agreed-upon currencies of sec-ondary reward, but what of its significance?

Damasio[10] has speculated that the emotions can be interpreted as a sys-tem for evaluating secondary reward. In an experiment involving two decks of cards, subjects can ask for a card from deck A or deck B. Deck A has a positive mean value but a low variance. In contrast, deck B has a neg-ative mean value but a high variance. Normal subjects experiment at first, picking cards from both A and B, but after they realize the statistical situ-ation, they stick to A. Subjects who have had a brain lesion in an area me-diating emotions stick with deck B despite its consequences. In addition, galvanic skin response, an electrical response indicating anxiety, can be measured in both groups. Normals reveal a response when reaching for B, indicating that internal mechanisms are registering the value of the choices, even before they can articulate their strategy! Damasio speculates that emotions, or "gut feel," are being used to evaluate choices. But we can go further in the light of data compression. Sensorimotor codes can be de-veloped to compress experience, but one wants to do better. Figure III.4 shows the problem. Suppose the light sensory situations are good and the grey ones are bad, but, based on their sensory codes alone, they are inter-mingled, thwarting attempts to encode them succinctly. Adding reward bits augments the state space, and changes the metric between these

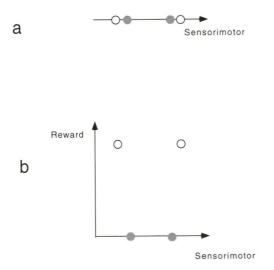

Figure III.4 (*a*) Data that have very different rewards, such as low (gray) or high (white), can have similar sensorimotor descriptions. (*b*) Adding reward bits changes the metric so that situations with similar reward are near each other.

choices. A mechanism that predicts basic reward values, like food, may have been co-opted to work for more abstract situations.

SYSTEM INTEGRATION

Evidence suggests that these different operations are in fact closely linked in momentary cognitive processing. In recent studies of Parkinson's patients, a disease associated with damage to the basal ganglia, patients performing a task very like the blocks task have revealed deficits in working memory.[11] Consider the interaction of vision and action. If the hippocampus[12] is the gateway that enables the retention of temporary visual information, and if a basal ganglia deficit produces a working memory deficit, the simplest implication is that this circuitry functions in a closed loop. This is understandable, as the basal ganglia represent motor program sequencing information, the visual cortex represents potential locations, and the hippocampus enables extracted locations to be saved in permanent memory. Thus the disparate purposes of similar actions can be resolved by the basal ganglia, which represent essential programmatic temporal context on "why" those actions are taking place and "when" they should be used. A specific example makes this point. Experiments in cortical area 46 have shown that there are memory representations for the next eye movement in motor coordinates.[13] However, this representation does not necessarily contain the information as to when it is to be used; that kind of information is part of a motor program such as might be found in the basal ganglia. For this reason the anatomical connections of the basal ganglia should be very important, as they may have to influence the sequencing of processing.

LEARNING MODELS

The learning models that are used to model programs at the 300-ms time-scale can be broadly characterized as *reinforcement learning* models. They have several distinct features.

1. Programs are modeled as a set of actions that are available for each of a set of discrete states.

2. The actions themselves are probabilistic.

3. The value of taking an action is signaled using a model of chemical reward. Reinforcement learning has a scalar reward that values each state in a behavioral program.

4. The technical problem of reinforcement learning, which is also experienced in biological systems, is that rewards are delayed.

The reinforcement learning algorithm itself finds sequences of actions to direct the physical system in the course of behavior. Most important, the mathematics required to do this is a direct descendant of the dynamic programming described in Section 6.4.2.

Markov Systems

The problem defined by any agent is not only to define a problem state space but also to define a model that expresses the transitions between different states. An extremely useful way of doing so that handles uncertainty is to allow probabilistic transitions between states. Such a system is called a *hidden Markov model*, or HMM. The use of the word "hidden" signifies that the real states of the world are not known, and that the model states are therefore estimates.

In building the HMM, the transitions through the network can be seen as analogous to the "control" signal in the optimal control formulation. Furthermore, the discrete nature of the model is ideally suited to dynamic programming, or DP. Thus DP-like algorithms are used to compute most probable paths through the network.

Reinforcement Learning

Hidden Markov models provide the necessary substrate for describing reinforcement learning. The big difference is that there are now actions that are under the control of the animal. These actions may have probabilistic outcomes, but in the same way that probabilistic outcomes in HMMs could be handled by the DP formalism, so can these probabilistic actions be handled by DP. Now the "control" signal is a reward that is associated with each action. Reinforcement learning adjusts the rewards associated with actions such that paths through the state space tend to maximize reward.

NOTES

1. A. Yarbus, *Eye Movements and Vision* (New York: Plenum, 1967).

2. Dana H. Ballard, Mary M. Hayhoe, and Jeff B. Pelz, "Memory Representations in Natural Tasks," *Journal of Cognitive Neuroscience* 7, no. 1 (1995):66–80; J. Grimes and G. McConkie, "On the Insensitivity of the Human Visual System to Image Changes Made During Saccades," in K. A. Akins, ed., *Problems in Perception* (Oxford: Oxford University Press, 1996); M. Tanenhaus, M. Spivey-Knowlton, K. Eberhard, and J. Sedivy, "Using Eye Movements to Study Spoken Language Comprehension: Evidence for Visually-Mediated Incremental Interpretation," in T. Inoui and J. McClelland, eds., *Attention and Performance XVI: Integration in Perception and Communication* (Cambridge, MA: MIT Press, 1995).

3. Both Strick and Hikosaka, independently, have shown this result: Peter L. Strick, Richard P. Dum, and Nathalie Picard, "Macro-Organization of the Circuits Connecting the Basal Ganglia with the Cortical Motor Areas," in James C. Houk, Joel L. Davis, and David G. Beiser, eds., *Models of Information Processing in the Basal Ganglia* (Cambridge, MA: MIT Press, Bradford, 1995, pp. 117–30); O. Hikosaka and R. Wurtz, "Visual and Oculomotor Functions of Monkey Substantia Nigra Pars Reticulata. III. Memory-Contingent Visual and Saccade Responses," *Journal of Neurophysiology* 49 (1983):1268–84; Hikosaka and Wurtz, "Visual and Oculomotor Functions of Monkey Substantia Nigra Pars Reticulata. IV. Relation of Substantia Nigra to Superior Colliculus," *Journal of Neurophysiology* 49 (1983):1285–1301.

4. Wolfram Schultz, Ranulfo Romo, Tomas Ljungberg, Jacques Mirenowicz, Jeffrey R. Hollerman, and Anthony Dickinson, "Reward-Related Signals Carried by Dopamine Neurons," in Houk, Davis, and Beiser, eds., *Models of Information Processing in the Basal Ganglia*, pp. 233–48.

5. Ibid.

6. Ben Pansky and Delmas J. Allen, *Review of Neuroscience* (New York: Macmillan, 1980), p. 275.

7. Ibid., p. 347.

8. Donald J. Woodward, Alexandre B. Kirillov, Christopher D. Myre, and Steven F. Sawyer, "Neostriatal Circuitry as a Scalar Memory: Modeling and Ensemble Neuron Recording," in Houk, Davis, and Beiser, eds., *Models of Information Processing in the Basal Ganglia*, pp. 315–36; Schultz et al., "Reward-Related Signals Carried by Dopamine Neurons"; Strick, Dum, and Picard, "Macro-Organization of the Circuits Connecting the Basal Ganglia with the Cortical Motor Areas."

9. M. A. Wilson and B. L. McNaughton, "Dynamics of the Hippocampal Ensemble Code for Space," *Science* 261 (1993):1055; J. O'Keefe and L. Nadel, *The Hippocampus as a Cognitive Map* (Oxford: Oxford University Press, 1978), pp. 150–53.

10. Antonio R. Damasio, *Descartes' Error: Emotion, Reason, and the Human Brain* (New York: G. P. Putnam, 1994).

11. John Gabrieli, "Contribution of the Basal Ganglia to Skill Learning and Working Memory in Humans," in Houk, Davis, and Beiser, eds., *Models of Information Processing in the Basal Ganglia*, pp. 277–94.

12. Recent work implicates the entorhinal cortex as the source of some of the effects previously associated with the hippocampus. Also, the hippocampus has a role in the transfer of short-term memory to long-term memory rather than being the source of the representation of STM. For the purposes of discussion, however, these very important points are details; it is necessary only that this general area be a necessary part of the total functioning of STM.

13. Patricia S. Goldman-Rakic, "Toward a Circuit Model of Working Memory and the Guidance of Voluntary Motor Action," in Houk, Davis, and Beiser, eds., *Models of Information Processing in the Basal Ganglia*, pp. 131-48.

10 Markov Models

ABSTRACT   A simple model of the brain's programs is the *Markov model*. In this model, transitions between states are probabilistic and depend only on the current state. A key representation of the state is in terms of its probability vector. A *regular* Markov process, where each of the states can be reached from each other, has a limiting probability vector that is an eigenvector of the transition matrix. For *nonregular* processes the transition matrix can be decomposed into regular and transient components. When the Markov process is an approximation of the world, it is said to be *hidden*. The key questions about hidden Markov models center on the degree to which they capture the essence of the underlying hidden process.

10.1 INTRODUCTION

This chapter describes a general way of composing look-up tables that is termed the *Markov model.* The Markov model uses discrete state spaces and probabilistic transitions between them.

To motivate this model, it helps to review the notions behind deterministic state spaces. In the eight-puzzle, the definition of the state space is unambiguous: The configuration of the board at any time corresponds to a unique state vector. Furthermore, in the model, the result of moving a tile is unambiguous: The tile cannot stick in an in-between place, so the transition to a new state is predictable. In the real world, however, the tile may stick, or the number on a tile may not be completely legible. This unpredictability in the real world makes it very natural for state changes in a model of that world to be probabilistic. Rather than being certain that a state change has occurred, the transition to a new state occurs with a certain probability. What should be the basis of choosing this probability? An extremely important class of models has the constraint that the probability of transiting to a new state depends only on the current state. This class is called Markov models.

Reliable state transitions and unambiguous states may still be a good model for the eight-puzzle, but it becomes more controversial as a model for chess (even though it is used by the best computer chess programs). The reason is that in the case of chess the literal description of states is very expensive, owing to the explosion of states that results from the enormous number of possible chess moves. What would really be useful would be to have a description of a state that captured the notion of the endgame, so

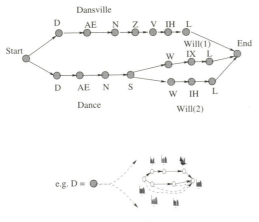

Detailed Model For a Phoneme

Figure 10.1 The use of Markov models in speech recognition. (*top*) The probability of a word such as "Dansville" may be computed from the probabilities of possible phoneme sequences. (*bottom*) The phoneme probabilities in turn may be computed from sequences of raw speech data features.

that one could implement the action "Near the endgame put the rooks on open files." For this we need a state space that is not literal, but instead summarizes key features of different world situations that call for a common response. This is the basis for *hidden Markov models*, which do not have access to the states of the world (they are, for one reason or another, "hidden"), and so create a Markov model that approximates the states of the world.

Markov models are widespread in speech recognition, as the speech data are very ambiguous, yet their interpretation depends on the surrounding context. Figure 10.1 illustrates the basic idea.

10.2 MARKOV MODELS

Given that a Markov model is one wherein the state transitions are probabilistic and the transition probabilities depend only on the current state, it is completely described by its transition matrix $A(t)$ where t is discrete. For each element $a_{ij}(t)$,

$$a_{ij}(t) = \text{probability of transiting from state } x_i(t) \text{ to state } x_j(t+1) \qquad (10.1)$$

Note that the columns of $a_{ij}(t)$ must sum to one. The transition matrix defined in Equation 10.1 allows for the transition probabilities to change as a function of time. However, a case of overwhelming utility is the *stationary* Markov process, wherein the transition matrix entries do not depend on time. The *order* of the Markov process is the number of states upon which the next state depends.

To simulate the Markov process, first pick a starting state x_0. Next pick a successor state according to the probabilities a_{0j} for $j = 1,..., N$. This will determine a new state x_1. Now repeat the process to generate the next state, and so on. Owing to the probabilistic nature of the model, every time this simulation is repeated a different sequence of states is likely to result. Thus the only way to analyze the process is to keep track of the probabilities of being in a state. Let

P_i = the probability that the Markov process is in state x_i

so that p is the state probability vector

$$p = \begin{pmatrix} P_1 \\ P_2 \\ \vdots \\ P_N \end{pmatrix}$$

The evolution of the probability vector is governed by the transition matrix; that is, the probabilities at time $t = 1$ are related to those at $t = 0$ by

$$p^T(1) = p^T(0)A$$

The probability vector $p^T(2)$ is similarly related to $p^T(1)$. Thus after t time steps,

$$p^T(t) = p^T(0)A^t$$

10.2.1 Regular Chains

Given that the probability vector $p^T(t)$ is evolving in time, it is natural to ask if there are circumstances in which there is an equilibrium probability distribution p^* such that

$$\lim_{t \to \infty} p(t) = p^*$$

It turns out that this can be answered for *regular* Markov processes.

A Markov process is said to be *regular* if for some n, $A^n > 0$.

For regular Markov processes, the limiting distribution is given by Theorem 10.1. This theorem is just a special case of the Frobenius-Perron theorem of Chapter 4. In fact, you can use the fact that the column sums bracket the eigenvalue to show that the eigenvalue must be one. Since all the rows are identical and they are probability vectors, they must all sum to one. Thus the upper and lower bound on λ is one.

Theorem 10.1

If a Markov process is regular, then there exists a unique probability vector **p** such that

1. $p^T A = p^T$

2. $\lim_{n \to \infty} A^n = A^*$, where A^* is composed of n identical rows equal to p^T.

Example To see that this approach works, consider the matrix A given by

$$A = \begin{bmatrix} .1 & .2 & .3 \\ .4 & .2 & .4 \\ .5 & .6 & .3 \end{bmatrix}$$

The product A^2 is given by

$$A^2 = \begin{bmatrix} .24 & .24 & .20 \\ .32 & .36 & .32 \\ .44 & .40 & .48 \end{bmatrix}$$

And the limit A^∞ is

$$A^\infty = \begin{bmatrix} .22 & .22 & .22 \\ .33 & .33 & .33 \\ .44 & .44 & .44 \end{bmatrix}$$

The maximum eigenvalue is one, as is seen by the column sums, which bracket it.

10.2.2 Nonregular Chains

In a regular transition matrix all the states are *accessible* from each other in that there is a finite-length path of nonzero probability between any two states. In the general case there will be states that are inaccessible from each other. States that are accessible from each other *communicate* with each other.

The states of a Markov process can always be divided into classes wherein the states in each class communicate only with other states from that class. Furthermore, the state of a finite Markov process will eventually enter a closed communicating class with probability one. A consequence of this is that the transition matrix of any nonregular Markov process can always be organized into four submatrices, as shown.

$$A = \begin{bmatrix} A_c & 0 \\ A_{tc} & A_t \end{bmatrix}$$

Here

1. The matrix A_c represents the accessible states and is regular, so that the results for regular processes apply.

2. The matrix A_t represents transitions among transient states.

3. The matrix A_{tc} represents transitions between transient and closed states.

10.3 HIDDEN MARKOV MODELS

Assume that a process in the world is Markovian but that its description is unknown. Then the task of the modeler is to define a Markov model that approximates the world process. This model is termed a hidden Markov model (HMM)[1] because the world process is hidden from the modeler. Consider a simple example where a person behind a screen is calling out the results of flipping a coin. The sequence of such flips is a set of *observations.* A result of a given set of eight flips might be

H H T H H T T H

The central question is, What model should be built to explain the observed sequences? A moment's reflection should convince you that there are many different answers to this question. One possibility is that a single coin is being used. But another possibility is that three coins are being used, and that flipping the first is used to select one of the remaining coins. Then the selected coin is flipped twice and its results reported. Given the preceding sequence it might be difficult to prefer the more complicated model over the simple, one-coin model. But if we were given the sequence

H H H H T T T T T T H H H H H T T H H H H

and were told that coins two and three were unfair, being biased toward heads and tails, respectively, then the second model would seem preferable. The goal of this section is to develop the formalism that allows one to choose between different Markov models.

10.3.1 Formal Definitions

A slightly richer process that will serve to flesh out the necessary formalisms is an urn model. Assume that there are N urns containing L colored balls, *Black, White,* and *Gray.* This is shown in Figure 10.2. A person starts at one of the urns, draws a ball and observes its color, replaces it, goes to another urn with a certain probability, and takes another ball. After T such drawings, the process ends.

The urn example contains all the elements that are needed to define an HMM:

1. A set of states x_i, $i = 1, \ldots, N$. In this case there are N states corresponding to the different urns. Let x denote the variable state vector and let s denote the specific set of states that would arise.

2. A set of observations b_j, $i = 1, \ldots, L$. In the example there are L observations corresponding to the different colors of the balls. While b denotes the variables, let O denote a specific set of observations that would result from an experiment.

3. A probability distribution for the start state:

$$\pi = \{\pi_i\}, \quad \text{where} \quad \pi_i = P(x_i^1)$$

4. A probability distribution for the state transitions:

$$A = \{a_{ij}\}, \quad \text{where} \quad a_{ij} = P(x_j^{t+1} \mid x_i^t)$$

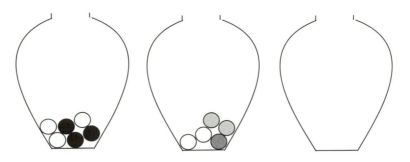

Figure 10.2 The urn model illustrates the basis of the hidden Markov model. A person randomly chooses an urn, draws a ball, and reports its color, repeating this process T times.

5. The probability distribution for the observations given the state:

$$B = \{b_j(k)\}, \quad \text{where} \quad b_j(k) = P(O_k \mid x_j)$$

The core of the model consists of the three probability distributions π, A, and B. Thus we can succinctly write the HMM as $M = (\pi, A, B)$. One way to use the model would be to "run" it and generate some sequences of observations, as shown in Algorithm 10.1.

To make things concrete, consider a specific configuration for the urns. Suppose there are two states, so that $N = 2$, and there are three observation times, so that $T = 3$. This model is shown in Figure 10.3.

Now choose the probability of the initial state as

$$\pi = \begin{pmatrix} .7 \\ .3 \end{pmatrix}$$

The matrix $b_j(k)$ defines the possible observations for each state. Pick

$$B = \begin{pmatrix} b_1(White) & b_1(Black) & b_1(Gray) \\ b_2(White) & b_2(Black) & b_2(Gray) \end{pmatrix}$$

$$= \begin{pmatrix} .1 & .4 & .5 \\ .6 & .2 & .2 \end{pmatrix}$$

Next we need a transition matrix A. Let's pick

$$A = \begin{bmatrix} .8 & .2 \\ .1 & .9 \end{bmatrix}$$

Algorithm 10.1   Generate Sequences

---

1. $t = 1$

2. Pick an initial state using π.

3. While $(t \le T)$ do the following:

a. Pick an observation O using B.
b. Pick a new state using A.
c. $t := t + 1$

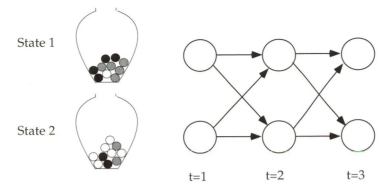

State 1

State 2

t=1   t=2   t=3

Figure 10.3 A specific urn model with two states that is used for three time steps. Each urn contains balls of three colors: black, white, and gray.

From this model and the algorithm for generating sequences, it is easy to guess that the most probable sequence would be *Gray, Gray, Gray*. Intuitively, this outcome occurs because state 1 is the most probable starting state, *Gray* is the most likely ball to be drawn from urn 1, and once drawing from urn 1, the most probable state is still urn 1. In a moment, we will verify this result formally.

10.3.2 Three Principal Problems

Now that the model is defined, you can use it to solve problems. There are three kinds of problems that can be addressed.

• **Problem 1: Find the probability of a given sequence of observations.** Solving this problem allows the comparison of different models. The best model is the one that has the highest probability of generating the observed sequences. In speech recognition, HMMs for different words compete against each other to explain the observed phoneme sequences. Alternate paths through each HMM are alternate ways of pronouncing a word. This problem is a form of maximum likelihood estimation. The data are the observations O and the model M is known. The task is to pick O to maximize

$$P(O \mid M)$$

• **Problem 2: Given a sequence of observations, find the most likely sequence of states in the model.** This state estimation problem is important in behavioral models. Earlier we saw that states can be defined deterministically with different kinds of memory models. But it may be the case that being absolutely sure of the state is too expensive and that the state can be defined much more economically in terms of the state sequence description. In this case it becomes important to have a method of estimating state sequence probabilities. This case can also be seen as a version of maximum likelihood. The task is

$$\max_{x^t} \left[\prod_{t=1}^{T} P(x_i^t \mid O, M) \right]$$

• **Problem 3: Adjust the model parameters to maximize** $P(O \mid M)$. This final problem addresses the design of the model itself. The best models will explain the observation sequences with the highest probabilities. It is difficult to do so, as the parameters that can be adjusted are all the parameters of the HMM.

$$\max_{M} [P(O \mid M)]$$

10.3.3 The Probability of an Observation Sequence

Solving the first problem turns out to be straightforward, since the probability of observing a given sequence $P(O \mid M)$ can be calculated directly. Let I be a particular sequence of states possible with the model; that is, $I = s_1, s_2, \cdots, s_T$. Observe that the $P(O \mid M)$ can be expanded simply summing over all possible state sequences. That is,

$$P(O \mid M) = \sum_{\forall I} P(O, I \mid M) \tag{10.2}$$

For any individual state sequence, one can use Bayes' rule to write $P(O, I \mid M)$ as

$$P(O, I \mid M) = P(O \mid I, M) P(I \mid M)$$

The first term on the right-hand side is simply the probability of seeing a given sequence of observations given a set of states. The known states allow its direct calculation as

$$P(O \mid I, M) = \Pi_{j \in I} b_{jk}(O_k)$$

Evaluating the second term is also simple, given a state sequence. It is the product of the probability of starting in state s_1 and traversing states $s_2, \ldots, s_T$:

$$P(I \mid M) = \pi_{i1} a_{s_1 s_2} a_{s_2 s_3} \cdots a_{s_{T-1} s_T}$$

The big drawback with this formulation is that summing over all the state sequences in Equation 10.2 is expensive, as there are on the order of N^T of them. Fortunately there is a better way, which uses partial results that accumulate in a vector $\boldsymbol{a}_t$. This is described by Algorithm 10.2.

Algorithm 10.2 Compute $P(O \mid M)$

1. $\boldsymbol{a}^1 = \boldsymbol{\pi} \otimes \boldsymbol{b}(O_1)$

2. For $t = 1, \ldots, T - 1$,

$\boldsymbol{a}^{t+1} = A[\boldsymbol{a}^t \otimes \boldsymbol{b}(O_{t+1})]$

3. $P(O \mid M) = \sum_{i=1}^{N} a_i^T$

To see how the efficient solution works, let's try it out on the urn model. The key is to define $\boldsymbol{\alpha}_i^t$ as the probability of seeing the observation O_{t+1} in state s_i given the previous history of observations. Then

$$\boldsymbol{\pi} = \begin{pmatrix} 0.7 \\ 0.3 \end{pmatrix} \quad \text{and} \quad \boldsymbol{b}(Gray) = \begin{pmatrix} 0.5 \\ 0.2 \end{pmatrix}$$

The initial vector $\boldsymbol{\alpha}^1$ is given by

$$\boldsymbol{\alpha}^1 = \begin{pmatrix} \pi_1 b_1(Gray) \\ \pi_2 b_2(Gray) \end{pmatrix} = \begin{pmatrix} .35 \\ .06 \end{pmatrix}$$

Next, $\boldsymbol{\alpha}^2$ is given by

$$\boldsymbol{\alpha}^2 = \begin{bmatrix} .8 & .2 \\ .1 & .9 \end{bmatrix} \begin{pmatrix} \alpha_1^1 b_1(Gray) \\ \alpha_2^1 b_2(Gray) \end{pmatrix} = \begin{pmatrix} .35 \\ .06 \end{pmatrix}$$

and $\boldsymbol{\alpha}^3$ is given by

$$\boldsymbol{\alpha}^2 = \begin{bmatrix} .8 & .2 \\ .1 & .9 \end{bmatrix} \begin{pmatrix} \alpha_1^2 b_1(Gray) \\ \alpha_2^2 b_2(Gray) \end{pmatrix} = \begin{pmatrix} .14 \\ .03 \end{pmatrix}$$

So that, finally, the probability of seeing the sequence *Gray, Gray, Gray* is given by

$$P(O \mid M) = \sum_{i=1}^{2} \alpha_i^3 = 0.17$$

As we have just seen, the key to the algorithm is the $\boldsymbol{\alpha}$s, which can be defined recursively, as shown in Figure 10.4. You may have recognized that the form of this algorithm is that of dynamic programming, introduced in Chapter 6.

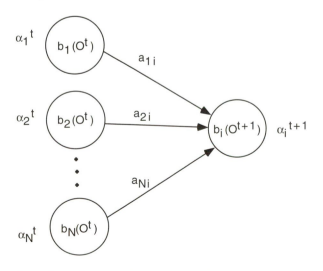

Figure 10.4 The recursive definition of the $\boldsymbol{\alpha}$s.

10.3 Hidden Markov Models

Algorithm 10.2 is known as the *forward* procedure, as it accumulates partial results going forward in time. In a completely analogous way one can define a backward procedure that starts at $t = T$ and ends at $t = 1$ (see Exercises). Let's assume for the moment that this procedure is followed and that we have vector $\boldsymbol{\beta}_t$ that keeps track of the probability of getting to one of the final states from the current state i. This $\boldsymbol{\beta}^t$ can be used to define an algorithm for predicting the probability of state sequences in an analogous way to the algorithm using $\boldsymbol{\alpha}$s (see Exercises).

10.3.4 Most Probable States

The problem of finding the optimal state sequence is underconstrained without some notion of optimality. A straightforward optimality criterion is the sequence that makes each of the states the most probable. A problem is that there might not even be a path between successor states determined this way, but in practice this difficulty rarely occurs. To express the solution, it helps to define γ_i^t as

$$\gamma_i^t = P(x_i^t = s_i \mid O, M)$$

Now γ^t can be expressed in terms of the $\boldsymbol{\alpha}$s and $\boldsymbol{\beta}$s, since

$$\gamma^t = \frac{\boldsymbol{\alpha}^t \otimes \boldsymbol{\beta}^t}{P(O \mid M)} \tag{10.3}$$

where $P(O \mid M)$ is a normalization factor so that $\sum_{i=1}^{N} \gamma_i^t = 1$. Thus γ_i^t is the probability of ending up in state s_i at time t, given the sequence of observations O. This can be factored into two parts: (1) the probability of ending up in state s_i at time t starting from a state at $t = 1$; and (2) the probability of starting from state s_i at time T and finishing up at some state at time T.

Given γ_i^t, the most probable states are easily expressed as

$$i_t = \mathrm{argmax}_{1 \leq i \leq N}[\gamma_i^t]$$

From Equation 10.3 it is easily seen that the computation can be done in two passes: one to calculate the $\boldsymbol{\alpha}$s and another to calculate the $\boldsymbol{\beta}$s. However, a one-pass algorithm, termed the Viterbi algorithm, can be found. To keep track of the best states, define an array r^t as shown in Algorithm 10.3.

Algorithm 10.3 Most Probable State Sequence

---

1. $\gamma_i^1 = \max_i \{\pi_i b_i (O_1)\}$

   $r(1) = i*$

2. For $t = 1, \ldots, T - 1$,

   $\gamma^{t+1} = \max_i \{a_{ij} [\gamma_i^t b_i (O_{t+1})]\}$

   $r(t) = i*$

Algorithm 10.3 works very similarly to its predecessor, except that the maximum is taken in place of the sum.

10.3.5 Improving the Model

The third problem in HMMs is to find the best model M. This turns out to be very difficult and has no known analytical solution. What can be done is to derive an approximation that is better than the current version. This procedure can be iterated until there is no further improvement. In outline, the strategy will be to start with an initial set of $M = (\pi, A, b)$ and run the model a sufficient number of times to estimate a new set of parameters $M' = (\pi', A', b')$. These estimates are then used as the new model, and the process is repeated. The estimates of π and b are simple.

$$\pi' = \gamma_t \tag{10.4}$$

$$b_j(k)' = \frac{\sum_{t=1, O_t=k}^{T} \gamma_t(j)}{\sum_{t=1}^{T} \gamma_t(j)} \tag{10.5}$$

The remaining task is to estimate a_{ij}. This can be done by defining the estimate η_{ij} as

$$\eta_{ij} = P(x_i^t = s_i, x_i^{t+1} = s_j \mid O, M)$$

Now η_{ij} can be written as

$$\eta_{ij} = \frac{\alpha_t(i) a_{ij} b_j(O_{t+1}) \beta_{t+1}(j)}{P(O \mid M)}$$

so that the estimate can be obtained from η_{ij} by averaging over time, as follows:

$$a'_{ij} = \frac{\sum_{t=1}^{T} \eta_{ij}}{\sum_{t=1}^{T} \gamma_t(j)} \tag{10.6}$$

With the expression for a'_{ij} the reestimation formulas are complete; the new estimate for the model is given by $M' = (\pi', A', b')$. This reasoning leads directly to Algorithm 10.4, a way of improving the model that makes successive reestimations of the model parameters until no further improvement results.

Algorithm 10.4 Baum-Welch Model Reestimation

Repeat the following steps until the improvements in the model parameters are less than some error tolerance:

1. Estimate π from Equation 10.4.

2. Estimate B from Equation 10.5.

3. Estimate A from Equation 10.6.

NOTE

1. The material on HMMs follows the review by L. R. Rabiner and B. H. Juang, "An Introduction to Hidden Markov Models," *IEEE ASSP Magazine* 3, no. 4 (January 1986):4–16.

EXERCISES

1. A Markov model can be a very simple model for the weather. Assume that the winter weather for a given area can be characterized by three states: (sunny, snowy, cloudy). If it is sunny, then there is a .7 probability that, on the next day, it will remain sunny; otherwise it will turn cloudy. If it is snowy, then there is a .5 probability that it will remain snowy and an equal chance that it will become sunny or cloudy. If it is cloudy, then there is a .25 probability that it will remain cloudy, and a .5 probability that it will become sunny.

a. Draw a *state transition diagram* that shows the states and arcs between them labeled with their transition probabilities.
b. Calculate the limiting probabilities of it being (sunny, snowy, cloudy).

2. Show that the board game Monopoly can be approximated as a Markov process. Simplify the game to derive a transition matrix. Find the equilibrium states, and use them to compute the relative values of each of the real estate properties.

3. Define alternate models for the coin-flipping experiment.

4. In an urn problem there are three urns with different numbers of four differently colored balls in each:

• urn 1: red(2), blue(2), green(3), and yellow(3)
• urn 2: red(3), blue(1), green(5), and yellow(1)
• urn 3: red(4), blue(4), green(0), and yellow(2)

The transition matrix A is given by

$$A = \begin{bmatrix} .1 & .2 & .3 \\ .4 + (-1)^t .2 & .2 & .4 + (-1)^{t+1} .2 \\ .5 & .6 & .3 \end{bmatrix}$$

and π is given by

$$\pi = \begin{bmatrix} .5 \\ .2 \\ .3 \end{bmatrix}$$

a. Compute the probability of seeing the sequence {*yellow, yellow, red, blue*}.
b. Compute the probability of the sequence {*urn1, urn1, urn3*} given observations {*yellow, blue, blue, red*}.

5. Test the Baum-Welch algorithm computationally by using the urn model in the previous problem to generate data that are used to refine estimates for M. Test the algorithm from different starting points.

6. Define a backward procedure that is analogous to the forward procedure but works from $t = T$ to $t = 1$. Use it with the two-urn example to compute the probability of the observation sequence *gray, gray, gray.*

7. The Baum-Welch algorithm can be viewed as a component of the expectation-maximization algorithm (EM) introduced in Chapter 4. Describe how this could be used within the EM context for the problem of identifying words as those having the most probable set of phoneme sequences.

11 Reinforcement Learning

ABSTRACT   Reinforcement learning models allow an agent to actively choose a decision policy based on explorations of the environment. When exploring a state space of uncertain rewards, an agent can learn what to do by keeping track of its state history and appropriately propagating rewards through the state space. The cost of reinforcement learning can be greatly reduced by having a teacher provide hints during the learning process. Reinforcement learning is termed a *Markov decision process* when the world and the agent's model of that world are identical. The more important case is when the state space is only *partially observable*. In this case the agent must decide what to do based on a description of the world that is necessarily incomplete.

11.1   INTRODUCTION

The Markov models of the previous chapter allow the description of processes in the world, but they are passive. They cannot model an agent's actions that change the world. That task requires an extension of the model to incorporate the different actions available to the agent. This extension is termed a *Markov decision process*, or *MDP*. A Markov decision process differs from an HMM in that actions, though they are stochastic, are chosen by the user.

MDPs incorporate the bookkeeping needed to keep track of user-controlled actions. Modeling such actions introduces three new factors. One is that the consequences of an action may not be known *a priori*. The second is that even when the consequences of an action are known, the value of taking that action is usually unknown. In these cases the value of an action must be discovered by experiment. Third, the value of an action is difficult to determine because the rewards for performing it are *delayed*. An example that illustrates all these complications is that of balancing an inverted pendulum attached to a moving cart (Figure 11.1). A controller must implement a control *policy* $u(t)$, $t = 0, 1, 2,...$, in order to keep the pendulum as vertical as possible. The strength of the pushing or pulling force $|u|$ is such that typically many applications are required to keep the pendulum balanced. The crucial points are as follows:

1. The model is unknown but must be discovered. The equations of motion are learned only by applying forces and observing their consequences.

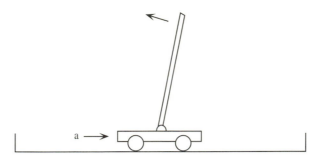

Figure 11.1 The cart and inverted pendulum problem. A cart moves on a one-dimensional track. Attached to the cart is a pendulum that is to be balanced. The control of the cart and pendulum is in the form of a discrete set of horizontal impulses $u = \pm a$ that are applied to the cart.

2. The utility of an action must also be learned by trying it out and seeing what happens.

3. The success or failure of the control policy is not known immediately, but only after the pole is horizontal or the cart hits the stop (failure), or when the pole is vertical (success).

The mathematics to handle delayed rewards is termed *reinforcement learning*. As emphasized in the introduction to this section, delayed rewards are a fundamental property of the world, and dealing with them successfully is vital to survival. Reinforcement learning does so in a direct way, creating a discrete state space that is a model for the world and then associating a *utility* for each state that reflects the possibility of getting a reward by taking actions from that state. The utility for each state is reminiscent of the heuristic function used to search state spaces in Chapter 3. The key difference between the algorithms used there and reinforcement learning is that the latter assumes that utility can be estimated using repeated trials. This assumption allows the cost of its estimation to be amortized over its useful lifetime.

Using this formalism, controllers for problems like the inverted pendulum can be designed. Section 11.2 describes how this designing is done. The example of maze following, in addition to the inverted pendulum balancing problem, is used to introduce the data structures that keep track of the calculations. Section 11.3 describes the core underlying mathematics behind reinforcement learning algorithms: the *policy improvement theorem*. This is the basis for the two reinforcement algorithms in most widespread use: *Q-learning* and *temporal difference learning*. The latter is the basis of a computer backgammon player that plays on a par with the best players in the world.

Reinforcement learning algorithms are expensive, and one way to dramatically reduce their cost is to use a *teacher*. This situation assumes that the reinforcement learning does not take place in isolation, but that there is an external source available for help. Formally, two extremes of teaching are (1) a critic and (2) a demonstrator. The first watches the performance of

Table 11.1 Categories of Markov models. Markov decision processes introduce an added layer of complexity by having control actions that are chosen by a learning algorithm.

	Passive	Active
Totally observable	Markov models	MDP
Partially observable	HMMs	PO-MDP

the agent and supplies only additional reward at crucial junctures. The second can only illustrate the problem solution by carrying out the individual steps. Very small amounts of such help can lead to dramatic improvements in performance.

Problems like the inverted pendulum are "small" problems in that the entire state space can be represented. For most problems the state space is too big. To handle this case, there must be a way of constructing an internal (hidden) Markov model that approximates the more complex external world. To distinguish this case, we term an MDP that uses an HMM a *partially observable MDP*. Table 11.1 shows how the HMM addition extends the modeling complexity.

The best way to build partial models is still an open problem. One approach is to try and avoid difficult parts of the state space where decisions are ambiguous. A simple problem of manipulating colored blocks illustrates this principle. Another approach is to act in the world and keep serial records of actions and rewards. After sufficient experience, these can be used to behave reliably.

11.2 MARKOV DECISION PROCESS

The essential feature of a Markov decision process is that the decision on the appropriate policy depends only on the current state. This allows complex processes to be modeled more simply, as only local interactions need be taken into account. In such a process, time is discrete. At each point in time the system occupies exactly one state. In that state, the agent executes an action that results in the receipt of a reward or penalty. At any time t,

- X_t is the random variable denoting the state of the system.
- x_t is the actual state of the system.
- R_t is the random variable denoting the reward received.
- r_t is the actual reward received.
- u_t is the action selected by the controller.

Remember that the crucial point is that the effects of an action depend only on the state in which it was performed. Thus the system is completely determined by a *transition function* $T(x_t, u_t) = X_{t+1}$ and an associated probability distribution $P_{xy}(u) = Pr[T(x, u) = y]$. The goal of a Markov decision process is to determine the expected reward for each state-action pair,

$\rho(x_t, u_t) = E(R_t)$. Once this determination has been made, a rational *policy* is to choose the actions that maximize reward.

Example 1: Maze Following   To see the computations involved, consider the very simple example of maze following shown in Figure 11.2. The problem is to learn a policy that will specify for each state the best action to move the agent toward the goal. The actions that the agent can use are to try to move in one of four compass directions, as shown in Figure 11.2. If there is a wall in that direction, the action has no effect, leaving the agent in the state (maze square) from which the action was taken. These effects for the example maze are shown in the transition function $T(x_t, u_t)$ in Table 11.2. The final part of the problem specification is the reward function:

$$R(x_t) = \begin{cases} 100 & x_t = 10 \\ 0 & \text{otherwise} \end{cases}$$

Table 11.2   The transition function for the maze problem.

	1	2	3	4	5	6	7	8	9	10
N	2	2	3	4	5	4	6	8	9	8
E	1	3	4	5	5	6	8	9	9	10
S	1	1	3	6	5	7	7	10	9	10
W	1	2	2	3	4	6	7	7	8	10

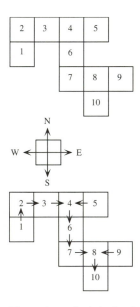

Figure 11.2   (*top*) A simple maze illustrates the mechanics of reinforcement learning. (*middle*) The transition function. For each state listed in the top row, the effects of the four possible actions are given in terms of the resultant state. (*bottom*) The optimal policy for the maze problem. From every state the arrow shows the direction in which to go in order to maximize reward.

The result of reinforcement learning is an optimal policy, shown in pictorial form in Figure 11.2 (*bottom*). The goal of a reinforcement learning algorithm is to calculate this policy.

Example 2: Pole Balancing   For the inverted pendulum and cart, the state is a four-dimensional vector

$$\mathbf{x}_t = \begin{pmatrix} x \\ \dot{x} \\ \theta \\ \dot{\theta} \end{pmatrix} \tag{11.1}$$

The control force on the cart is given by

$$u = \pm K$$

and the reward is given by the function

$$r = \begin{cases} +A & \theta = 0° \\ -B & \theta = 90° \quad \text{or} \quad x = 0 \quad \text{or} \quad x = L \end{cases}$$

To simulate the cart and pendulum motion, one must integrate the equations of motion, which are complicated,[1] being given by

$$\ddot{\theta} = \frac{g \sin \theta + \cos \theta \left(\dfrac{-u - ml\dot{\theta}^2 \sin \theta + \mu_c \, \mathrm{sgn}(\dot{x})}{m_c + m} \right) - \dfrac{\mu_p \dot{\theta}}{ml}}{l \left(\dfrac{4}{3} - \dfrac{m \cos^2 \theta}{m_c + m} \right)}$$

and

$$\ddot{x} = \frac{u + ml\dot{\theta}^2 \sin \theta - \ddot{\theta} \cos \theta + \mu_c \, \mathrm{sgn}(\dot{x})}{m_c + m}$$

Although these equations are complex, keep in mind that their complexity must be dealt with only in simulating their effects. In the real world, the world itself "runs" these equations to produce their effects, which are observed by the agent's sensors.

To set up the problem a memory is chosen by sampling the four dimensions of the state space. The result of reinforcement learning in this case is to find the appropriate control, either K or $-K$, for each point in the state space.

11.3   THE CORE IDEA: POLICY IMPROVEMENT

Reinforcement learning works because it is possible to make local improvements. At every point in the state space, the Markov property allows actions to be chosen based only on knowledge about the current state and the states reachable by taking the actions available at that state.

The policy updates are done in a manner similar to dynamic programming (introduced in Chapter 6). The difference is that dynamic programming normally takes one pass backward through the state space. Given terminal state and control, the system dynamics tell us what the previous state must have been. In contrast, in reinforcement learning, iterations are necessary to learn the control policy because the dynamics of the system are not known but must be learned by forward experiments. The only way to find out what happens in a state is to pick a control, execute it, and see where you end up. Doing it this way is possible because the iterative mechanism of dynamic programming works even when the policy and knowledge about the dynamics are only partially specified. To prove this statement formally requires a discussion of the *policy improvement theorem*.

The policy improvement theorem requires a formal specification of a policy and an additional bookkeeping mechanism to keep track of the value of states and actions. Figure 11.3 depicts the basic notation. Let $f(x)$ be the policy for every state x. The policy is simply the action to take in state x. Denote $V_f(x)$ as the value of the policy. This is the expected reward for following policy f from state x. Now let $Q(x, u)$ be the *action-value* function, or Q-function, for policy f. This is the expected return of starting in state x, taking action u, and then following policy f thereafter. The value function is related to the Q-function by

$$V_f(x) = \max_u [Q(x, u)]$$

In other words, the value of a state is the value of the best action available from that state. Thus it is easy to calculate V from Q. The next section shows how to calculate the Q-function itself.

The use of the Q-function allows the succinct formulation of the policy improvement theorem (see Box 11.1). The policy improvement theorem indicates that incrementally changing the policy to the action that is locally best is also the right global thing to do. This allows the development of local learning algorithms, such as Q-learning.

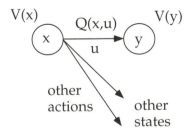

Figure 11.3 The basic vocabulary for reinforcement learning algorithms. The value function V rates each state. The action-value function $Q(x, u)$ rates the value of taking action u from state x.

Box 11.1   Policy Improvement Theorem

> Let f and g be chosen so that
>
> $Q[x, g(x)] \geq V_f(x)$
>
> Then
>
> $V_g(x) \geq V_f(x)$
>
> **Informal Proof:** If $Q[x, g(x)] \geq V_f(x)$, it means that it is better to follow g for one step and then follow f. However, by induction, it's also better to follow g for one more step and then follow f, and so on. So it's always better to pick g.

11.4   Q-LEARNING

At this point there is one thing left to do, and that is to compute the Q-values. To do so requires a way of estimating the value of actions. The value of actions that have immediate reward is easy; just use the reward itself as the value. The key decision concerns the weighting of future rewards. A reasonable way of valuing future rewards that makes the mathematics particularly simple is to use a discount factor that weights such rewards less and less exponentially. That is, where $t = 0$ is the present, use

$$\sum_{t=0}^{n} \gamma^t r_t \tag{11.2}$$

with $0 \leq \gamma \leq 1$.

The attraction of using a discount factor between zero and one is that algorithms such as Q-learning can be shown to converge.

The arguments so far use *estimates* of the discounted return. How are these estimates to be obtained? One way is to compute the value of specific actions on the fly in the course of doing experiments. As the action-value function $Q(x, u)$ is at the core of the estimation, the method is known as Q-learning. This learning can be further qualified by the temporal window used in the estimate of reward, Equation 11.2. *One-step* Q-learning uses $n = 1$ in this formula. Thus an estimate for the value of an action taken from a state x is given by

$$Q^{new}(x, u) = r + \gamma Q^{old}[x, f(x')]$$

where x' is that state that results from the execution of action u in state x. It turns out that a slightly better strategy is to use a weighted average between this estimate and the previous value.[2] This procedure results in

$$Q^{new}(x, u) = \eta Q^{old}(x, u) + (1 - \eta)\{r + \gamma Q^{old}[x, f(x')]\}$$

The complete algorithm is given as Algorithm 11.1. In that algorithm specification, step 2—"Select an action a to execute that is usually consistent with f but occasionally an alternate"—requires some elaboration. Early in the exploration phase, the estimates for Q will not be very accurate

Algorithm 11.1 One-Step Q-Learning Algorithm

Initialize $Q(x, u)$ as follows:

$f(x) := a$ such that $Q(x, a) = \max_u Q(x, u)$

Repeat the following until the policy converges:

1. Set x = current state.

2. Select an action a to execute that is usually consistent with f but occasionally an alternate.

3. Execute a and record the next state y and the reward r.

4. Update Q:

$Q^{new}(x, u) = (1 - \eta)Q^{old}(x, u) + \eta\{r + \gamma Q^{old}[x', f(x')]\}$

5. Update the policy

$f(x) := a$ such that $Q(x, a) = \max_u Q(x, u)$

owing to limited samples, so one would not want to get in a rut by picking a policy that is not significantly better (in the statistical sense). Unfortunately, it is not known exactly what the best exploration policy is. Only in the case that the rewards are fixed is the right policy known; this case has been formalized as the "k-armed bandit problem" and is discussed in Chapter 12 (Section 12.2.2) in a different context. There the solution is that if you have evidence that one choice is better than another, then you should sample that choice an exponentially increasing number of times. (You don't pick it exclusively on the increasingly remote chance that your samples are skewed.) However, in the current context, which has *shifting* rewards, there is only a heuristic sense that you should explore initially and then gradually become more biased toward the best policy. One such strategy can be expressed as follows: Pick the best action with probability

$P = 1 - e^{-an}$

where n is the number of samples and α is a parameter.

It is important to realize that this kind of exploration policy is consistent with the overlying principle of minimizing entropy! The entropy of a policy can be expressed in terms of the usual $\sum P_i \log P_i$, where P_i is the probability of a given path through a segment of the state space. As the policy becomes increasingly set, then the probability of one particular path through the state space will predominate, and the entropy will tend to zero.

11.5 TEMPORAL-DIFFERENCE LEARNING

The Q-learning algorithm works well but has a big drawback owing to its dynamic programming core. Since the experiments are being done in a forward manner and reward is propagating backward, a lot of early experiments are wasted. Initially only the penultimate moves have much effect. It would be nice if the earlier states were able to do something constructive while waiting for reward. One thing to do would be to record the results of the experiments in the form of a stochastic dynamics. In this way when the state function makes contact with reward, that reward can be "pushed back" using the dynamic equations in reverse. An alternate method, which is the subject of this section, is to have the system trying to make consistent predictions in the meantime. This is called temporal-difference learning.[3]

The best way to understand temporal-difference learning is to examine its learning rule. The setting is that of a feedforward network that is trying to estimate the value function. In other words, given the set of actions a_t available at time t, the right thing to do is to test them and record the resultant state y. Each of the new states is evaluated in turn using the network, and the one that produces the highest estimate of reward dictates the action that is chosen to move forward in state space. In following this procedure the network learns, for each state y, to produce an estimate of the value function V_t. This estimate in turn can be used to modify the network. The way this modification is achieved is to change the network's output unit weights according to

$$\Delta w = \eta (r_t + \lambda V_{t+1} - V_t) \sum_{k=1}^{k=t} \lambda^{t-k} \frac{\partial V_k}{\partial w}$$

where λ is a parameter that can range between 0 and 1 and η is a learning rate parameter that must be handpicked. To understand how this method might work, consider the case for λ very small. In this case only the $k = t$ term counts, and the formula reduces to

$$\Delta w = \eta (r_t + \lambda V_{t+1} - V_t) \frac{\partial V_t}{\partial w}$$

This is just a version of the backpropagation rule where the desired state is V_{t+1}. Thus the network is doing a "smoothing" operation that tries to make successive states make consistent predictions. Where there is actual reward, then the actual reward is used instead of the predicted reward. Thus the network works just like Q-learning. Reward centers provide concrete centers that propagate back to more distal states. You can show formally that any value of λ between 0 and 1 works, but that proof is too involved to be presented here.[4]

The complete algorithm is given as Algorithm 11.2.

Example: Backgammon   An interesting example in which temporal-difference learning works well is the game of backgammon. This is a board game in which opponents have 15 checkers that move in opposite directions along a linear track. Figure 11.4 shows a version of the standard backgammon board. The player with the black checkers must move them

Algorithm 11.2 Temporal Difference (TD) Algorithm

Initialize the weights in the network to random values. Repeat the following until the policy converges:

1. Apply the current state to the network and record its output V_t.

2. Make the move suggested by the network, and roll the dice again to get a new state.

3. Apply the new state to the network and record its output V_{t+1}. If the state is a win, substitute $V_{t+1} = 1$; if it's a loss, substitute $V_{t+1} = -1$.

4. Update the weights:

$$\Delta w = \eta(r_t + \lambda V_{t+1} - V_t) \sum_{k=1}^{k=t} \lambda^{t-k} \frac{\partial V_k}{\partial w}$$

5. If there are hidden units, then use Algorithm 8.1 to update their weights.

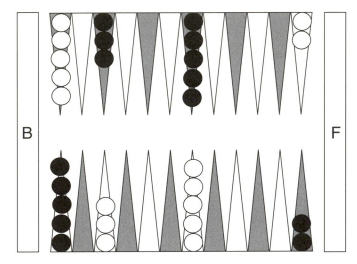

Figure 11.4 The backgammon board in its initial configuration. Opponents have checkers of a given color that can reside on the points shown as triangles. Players alternate turns. A turn consists of a roll of the dice and an advancement of checkers according to the dice roll.

clockwise from the position at the lower right toward the position at the upper right, and finally off the board. The player with the white checkers moves in the opposite direction. The movement of the checkers is governed by the roll of two dice.

Figure 11.5 shows a possible position in the middle of the game. Player 1, with the black checkers, has just rolled (6, 3). There are several options for playing this move, one of which is shown. Player 2 has a checker on the bar and must attempt to bring it onto the board on the next move. The game ends when all of one player's checkers have been "borne off," or removed from the board. At any time a player may offer to double the stakes of the game. The opposing player must either agree to play for

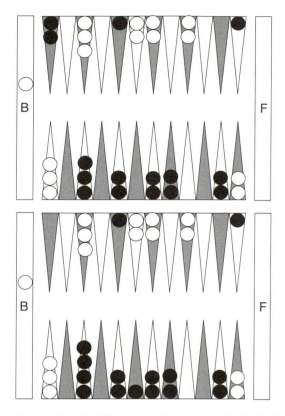

Figure 11.5 (*top*) Player 1, black, has just rolled (6, 3). (*bottom*) There are several options for playing this move, one of which is shown.

double stakes or forfeit the game. If the player accepts, then that player has the same option at a later time.

The backgammon network (Figure 11.6) consists of 96 units for each side to encode the information about the checkers on the board. For each position and color, the units encode whether there are one, two, three, or greater than three checkers present. Six more units encode the number of checkers on the bar and off the board, and the player to move, for a total of 198 units. In addition, the network uses hidden units to encode whole-board situations. The number of hidden units used ranges from none to 40.

It is interesting to inspect the features of the network after training, as they reveal the codes that have been selected to evaluate the board. For example, Figure 11.7 (*right*) shows large positive weights for black's home board points, large positive weights for white pieces on the bar, positive weights for white blots, and negative weights for white points on black's home board.[5] These features are all part of a successful black attacking strategy. Figure 11.7 (*left*) exhibits increasingly negative weights for black blots and black points, as well as a negative weighting for white pieces off and a positive weight for black pieces off. These features would naturally be part of an estimate of black's winning chances.

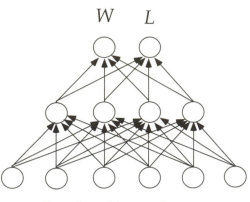

Board position and move

Figure 11.6 The architecture of the network used to estimate reward for backgammon.

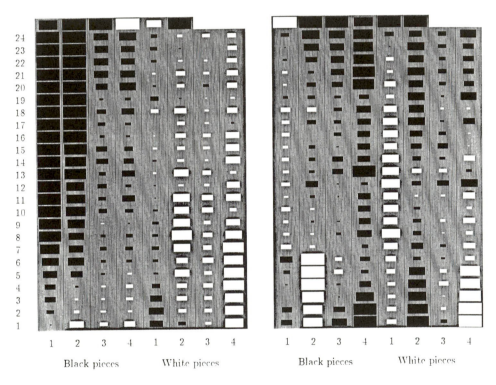

Figure 11.7 The weights from two hidden units after training. Black squares represent negative values; white squares, positive values. The size of the square is proportional to the magnitude of the weight. Rows 1–24 represent the 24 positions on the board. The top row represents (from right to left): white pieces on the bar, black pieces on the bar, white pieces borne off, black pieces borne off, white's turn, and black's turn. (Reprinted from Tesauro, 1992, *Machine Learning*, © 1992, with kind permission from Kluwer Academic Publishers.)

11.6 LEARNING WITH A TEACHER

The biggest speedup of all is to be told what to do. Learning agents do not learn in a vacuum but get much of their knowledge from others. It might seem that incorporating this knowledge into learning algorithms would be easy, but it is not. The difficulty is that the other agent has to communicate the knowledge successfully. If the two agents were copies of each other, communicating might be easy, but more realistically they have to communicate through a symbol system that is ambiguous. Nonetheless, teaching is effective.

This section describes the effectiveness of two simple teaching models that assume different properties of the teaching procedure. In the first, *learning with an external critic,* the teacher can correct the student by watching the student's actions and providing appropriate external reward. In the second, *learning by watching,* the student watches the teacher perform the behavior. In this case the actions are known, but the associated reward is not. The main point is that just a few of the appropriate signals are surprisingly effective.

Learning with an External Critic   Learning with an external critic (LEC) is modeled by converting a YES/NO signal from the teacher into an internal reward signal according to

$$
r_c(t) = \begin{cases} R_c & \text{if YES} \\ -R_c & \text{if NO} \\ 0 & \text{otherwise} \end{cases}
$$

This reward can be added to the Q-value and used to select subsequent actions. Another way reward can be used is to negatively reward inconsistent states. A state can be considered inconsistent if either

$Q(x, u) < 0$ and   YES

or

$Q(x, u) > 0$ and   NO

Figure 11.8 shows that just a little correction is sufficient to provide a large increase in performance.

Learning by Watching   Learning by watching (LBW) is modeled by having the agent use an internal switch. When the switch is in the "act" position, the agent learns using a standard Q-learning algorithm. But when the switch is in the "observe" position, the agent interprets a stream of the teacher's state action pairs. These pairs are used to update a bias function as follows: Internal state-action pairs that agree with the external decisions have their reward increased; and internal state-action pairs that do not match the teacher's decisions are decreased.

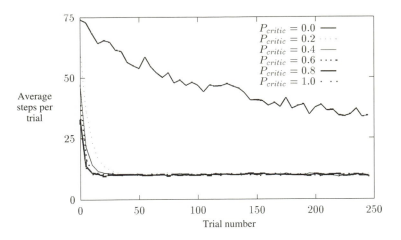

Figure 11.8 Learning with an external critic. P_{critic} is the probability that the critic will tell the agent the correct value of the action taken at each step. If there is just a small chance that the agent will be told the value of the action taken, learning is speeded up dramatically. (From Whitehead, 1992.)

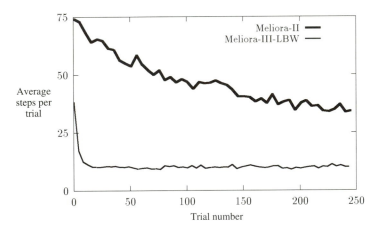

Figure 11.9 Learning by watching. In this paradigm the agent sees the correct actions taken, but has to learn their value. (From Whitehead, 1992.)

Figure 11.9 shows that just a little correction is sufficient to provide a large increase in performance.

An Abstract Model of Teaching Both the learning-by-criticism and learning-by-watching paradigms lead to dramatic speedups. Is there any way that we can appreciate these advantages in the abstract? One way is to model general learning as a random walk in a multidimensional state space.[6] The time to find reward can be calculated assuming that, at each step, the probability that the agent is heading toward the goal is a constant. Under these circumstances the effects of even modest progress are huge, as shown in Figure 11.10. The numbers show the probability, at each step, that the agent is moving *away* from the goal. If this is just slightly above

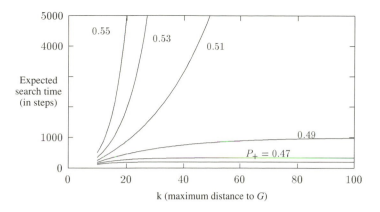

Figure 11.10 A small bias in a random walk has huge effects. Plotted is the expected time to get to the goal as a function of the distance to the goal. (From Whitehead, 1992.)

one-half, then the time to get there becomes exponential, whereas if it is just slightly below one-half, the time becomes sublinear.

11.7 PARTIALLY OBSERVABLE MDPs

In all the previous examples, the entire state space was observable. More generally, with complex worlds, representing them in their entirety would result in huge state spaces. Under these circumstances one is forced to try to represent just the important part of the state space relevant to the behavior. This is no easy task.

What happens when all the states cannot be represented depends on the perceptual apparatus. It could be the case that a large part of the world is not represented at all but that certain states are known exactly. Far more likely, however, is that the perceptual apparatus confuses states just as a color-blind person can confuse red and green. In this case we say that states are *perceptually aliased.* The idea is that the sensor does not have enough precision to distinguish them. A simple example illustrates the trouble this lack of precision causes. Suppose that the world consists of just eight states in a line with a reward at one end, as shown in Figure 11.11. In this problem, the optimal policy is to go right from any state. Now suppose that the perceptual apparatus of the agent is such that states 2 and 5 cannot be distinguished. The agent may be color-blind, for example. In this example the confounding of two states results in the wrong policy. State 25 in the model is sometimes world state 2 and sometimes world state 5. But when it is 5 the agent gets a large reward for going left, with the result that 25 is overvalued for the case when the agent is in state 2. Thus the decision is always "go left" from model state 3, which is always the wrong thing to do. Therefore, the correct policy cannot be learned.[7]

This section develops two ways of handling this problem. The more primitive is to recognize bad states and remove them from the model, and

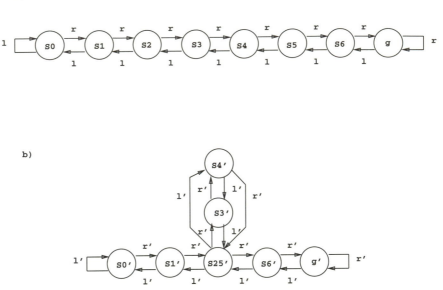

Figure 11.11 (*a*) A linear state space. (*b*) Its internal representation: States in the world are not distinguished internally, resulting in the topology shown. (Adapted from Whitehead and Ballard, 1991, *Machine Learning*, © 1991, with kind permission from Kluwer Academic Publishers.)

thus from consideration in the Q-learning algorithm. This would not work in the present example, owing to the paucity of states, but in a larger problem, the state space should be populated with alternate routes.

The more elegant solution to the perceptual aliasing problem is to expand the state space descriptions until they are unambiguous. This procedure must be carried out with care, as the cost of searching is an exponential function of the space. The method of utile distinctions[8] seeks to perform this task economically.

11.7.1 Avoiding Bad States

Consider the simple blocks world domain shown in Figure 11.12, and suppose that the task is very simple: pick up the green block. Representing the possible worlds with just configurations of 20 blocks results in over 40 billion states. Needless to say, searching these is impractical.

A way to start to fix this problem is to allow the sensory system the ability to represent just parts of the world at each moment. Suppose that the decision process is anthropomorphic and has two "windows" on the world. One could be the part of the world that is being directly looked at, and the other could be the part of the world that is being attended to. These are termed *markers*.[9] Markers represent the properties of blocks in the world momentarily, as shown by Figure 11.13. The point is that MDP has to use just the information related to the marked objects in

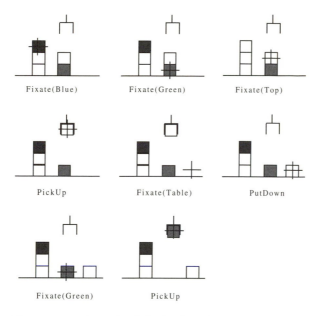

Figure 11.12 A graphical display from the output of a program that has learned the "pick up the green block" task. The steps in the program use deictic references rather than geometrical coordinates. For each stage in the solution, the plus symbol shows the location of the fixation point. (Adapted from Whitehead and Ballard, 1991, *Machine Learning*, © 1991, with kind permission from Kluwer Academic Publishers.)

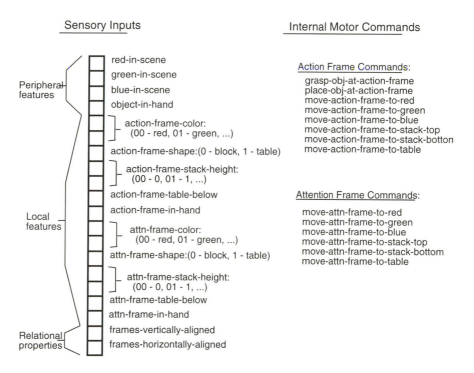

Figure 11.13 A state in the blocks world and its internal representation. (Adapted from Whitehead and Ballard, 1991, *Machine Learning*, © 1991, with kind permission from Kluwer Academic Publishers.)

making a decision. When the markers change position, the internal state changes also.

From the earlier example one might suspect that perceptual aliasing would play a role here, and it does, as shown by Figure 11.14. The figure shows states that are identical internally yet require different actions, owing to the surrounding context. One way to solve this difficulty is to try to avoid aliased states. Such states can be discovered if the process is deterministic, as they will exhibit a wide variance in their reward. Thus the standard Q-learning algorithm can be modified to incorporate the tracking of the variance of reward for all states. High-variance states can be directly devalued. The hope is that there are alternate unaliased sequences of actions that will solve the problem.

The elimination of high-variance states is a very crude way of attacking the perceptual aliasing problem, and there are a number of methods for making more refined decisions. The gist of these methods is to expand the state space by introducing additional elements into the state space description. As mentioned earlier, expanding the state space is extremely costly, so additional states must be introduced with care. To that end, these algorithms test the current state description against a proposed expanded description to see which is better. As the environment is usually stochastic, these tests are statistical in nature and, as a consequence, take the time needed to gather sufficient statistics. The cost of testing for splitting an ambiguous state into two less-aliased states can be significant. Two ways of splitting a state are (1) to make decisions based on an expanded perceptual description of the state[10] and (2) to make a decision based on the utility of the split versus unsplit situations.[11]

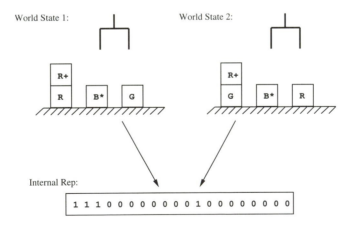

Figure 11.14 Perceptual aliasing in the blocks world example. Both of the situations have the same internal state owing to the way markers work. (Consult Figure 11.13 to interpret the state bits.) However, the correct actions are different. On the left, the next action is Fixate(Green) in preparation for picking up the green block. On the right, the next action is PickUp to clear off the top of the green block in preparation for picking it up. (Adapted from Whitehead and Ballard, 1991, *Machine Learning*, © 1991, with kind permission from Kluwer Academic Publishers.)

11.7.2 Learning State Information from Temporal Sequences

Another way to avoid the problem of perceptual aliasing is to augment the state information until each state is no longer ambiguous. The problem is that if this procedure is done haphazardly, the state space can quickly become too large. What one would like is a way of testing the state space so that it is just as large as it has to be. One way is to rely on real-world experience. When faced with making a decision, interrogate a library of previous experiences in which similar situations came up, and make the consensus decision. This method is shown in Algorithm 11.3. The library is built by recording the agent's experience as a sequence of states

$$x_i, i = 1, \ldots, t$$

where t is the current time. Associated with each state is the triple o_t, a_t, r_t denoting, respectively, the observation in state x_t, the action taken, and the reward received. In the earlier formulation, there are several actions possible from each state, and each has an associated Q-value. Here, the principal data structure is the record of what actually happened with one action per state. Thus there is only one Q-value, q_i, per state.

To understand how the algorithm works, consider the analogy with a k-nearest neighbor strategy, as shown in Figure 11.15.[12] In that strategy, to decide what to do in a given state, the k nearest neighbors in state space are interrogated. The states are represented abstractly as points in a hypothetical state space. Associated with each such point will be a policy. In the figure $k = 3$, and the three closest neighbors are indicated with shading. The action taken is a function of their policies; for example, the most frequent action may be taken. The k-nearest sequence strategy works similarly. The agent's history is examined for the k most similar temporal state trajectories. Here again $k = 3$, and the three most similar sequences are indicated with brackets. The chosen policy is a function of the policies recommended by the leading state in those sequences.

As shown in Figure 11.16, the k-nearest sequence algorithm can lead to dramatic performance improvements.

Algorithm 11.3 Nearest Sequence Memory

---

1. For each of the current actions, examine the history, and find the k most similar sequences that end with that action.

2. Each of these sequences will end in a state with an action. Each state votes for that action.

3. Compute the new Q-value by averaging the values for the successful voters.

4. The action with the most votes may be selected, or a random action (for exploration) may be selected.

5. Execute the action, recording the new state, together with its observation and reward.

6. Update the new Q-values.

Learning in a Geometric Space

k-nearest neighbor, *k* = 3

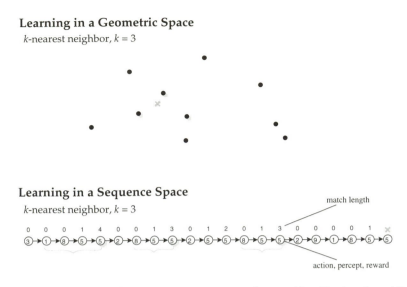

Learning in a Sequence Space

k-nearest neighbor, *k* = 3

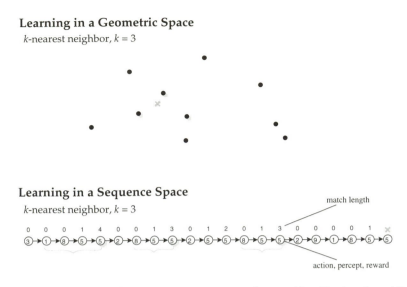

Figure 11.15 Using *k*-nearest sequence memory for state identification. (*upper*) In *k*-nearest neighbor the action to take in a given situation is determined from the actions stored in similar states, where similarity is determined from the state space encoding. (*lower*) In *k*-nearest sequence a record of the agent's history is kept. To determine the action to take at the current time, as indicated by the "x," the *k* closest sequences are determined from the history, and their actions are used to choose the current action. (From McCallum, 1995a. © MIT.)

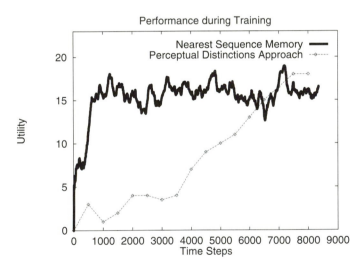

Figure 11.16 The *k*-nearest sequence algorithm can lead to significant speedups. Here it is compared to the Chrisman algorithm for resolving aliasing by adding perceptual bits. The graph shows roughly an order of magnitude in the time to converge to a high-utility policy. (From McCallum, 1995a. © MIT.)

11.7.3 Distiguishing the Value of States

The idea behind using temporal sequences to make decisions is simple on the surface: if there is a set of previous histories that resulted in a common action, then take that action this time as well. However, there is a subtlety to consider: how long should the sequence be? It could be the case that sequences that are short have higher utility than longer sequences, or vice versa. Guessing the sequence length based only on matches between the state action values in the absence of utility can lead to suboptimal decisions. A way around this difficulty is to let utility guide the selection of the sequence lengths. The goal is to partition the set of temporal sequences into subsets that have the same utility.

One way of creating these partitions is to use a tree to store the temporal sequences.[13] The tree consists of alternating levels, starting with the most recent observations, then the actions that led to those observations, next the observations that were obtained in the penultimate states, and so on. A representative tree for a hypothetical problem that has two possible actions and two possible observations is shown in Figure 11.17. The tree has two parts, one upon which the current policy is going to be based and another that stores longer sequences that are potential extensions to the current policy. The latter part is termed a *fringe* and is represented by the dotted lines in the figure.

A sequence of observations and actions accesses the current policy. For example, given 0 b 1, the current best action is stored at the leaf of the tree indicated by the arrow in Figure 11.17.

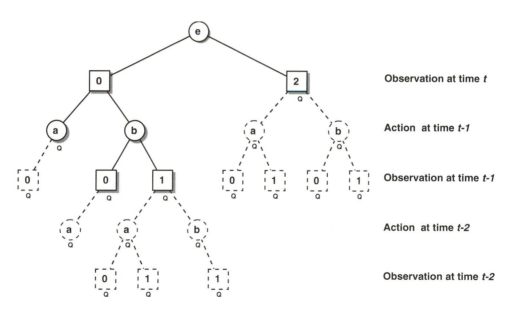

Figure 11.17 The tree data structure for indexing into temporal sequences. Percepts are indicated by integers, actions by letters. The fringe nodes are drawn in dashed lines. Nodes labeled with a Q are nodes that hold Q-values. (From McCallum, 1995b. © MIT.)

The fringe is used to check that longer sequences might not result in decisions that are better still. To do this checking one can test the value of a sequence against the penultimate sequence of shorter length. If the longer sequence makes useful distinctions, then that sequence is used as a baseline, and even longer sequences are represented in the fringe. This procedure is followed when taking an action generates a new observation of the state, resulting in a new temporal sequence which is then stored in the tree. For example, given the sequence

```
0 b 1 a
```

a test would be made to see if the tree should be extended to make the distinction between that and

```
0 b 1 b
```

or whether the current partition

```
0 b 1
```

should be kept as is.

The sequences are being used to define the state space incrementally. Each node in a leaf of the tree represents a state in the state space, and the agent is learning a policy that when executed will put it in another state that will also be a leaf node. The information in fringe nodes represents potential refinements of the state space. Thus the tree also guides the updating of the policy *values*.

To make these ideas more specific requires some definitions.

• An *instance* at time t is a four-tuple consisting of the previous instance, the action taken from that instance, and the observation and the reward received as a result of the action; that is,

$$T_t = \langle T_{t-1}, u_{t-1}, o_t, r_t \rangle$$

Stringing together the set of instances results in the temporal sequence used in the previous section.

• A *state* of the agent's model is represented as a leaf node of the *history tree*. This is explicitly denoted by referring to the transition that is stored in the leaf; that is,

$$x = L(T)$$

• The set of all instances that is associated with the leaf x is referred to by

$$T(x)$$

The ultimate goal of this version of reinforcement learning is of course to calculate a policy that specifies the action to be taken in each state. To rate the value of different actions, the Q-value iteration algorithm is used, with the updating determined by the appropriate partitions as captured by the tree. That is,

$$Q(x, u) \leftarrow R(x, u) + \gamma P(x' \mid x, u) U(x')$$

where $R(x, u)$ can be estimated as the average amount of reward obtained when action u was taken from state x,

$$R(x, u) = \frac{\sum_{T_i \in \mathcal{T}(x, u)} r_i}{|\mathcal{T}(x, u)|}$$

and the probability $P(x' \mid x, u)$ can be similarly estimated as the number of times taking u from x resulted in state x' in the partition divided by the total number of times u was chosen, or

$$P(x' \mid x, u) = \frac{|\forall T_i \in \mathcal{T}(x, u) \text{ s.t. } L(T_{i+1}) = x'|}{|\mathcal{T}(x, u)|}$$

Example: Hallway Navigation The use of a tree to index sequences of the same utility is illustrated with a simple example of searching a hallway to find a reward. In this case, as shown in Figure 11.18, the reward is the state labeled G at a central location. The agent has actions for moving along the compass directions of north, south, east, and west. What makes the problem partially observable is that the sensory information does not uniquely identify a state but only provides information as to local barriers in each of the four directions. Thus the code on the squares in the figure indicates the local surround. Positions that have the same configuration of surrounding walls get the same code. The agent receives a reward of 5.0 for reaching the goal, -1.0 for bumping into a wall, and -0.1 otherwise. For this example, the discount factor γ is 0.9, and the exploration probability is a constant 0.1.

Algorithm 11.4 is applied to this case, and the resultant tree that is built is shown in Figure 11.19. You can see that where the decision of which direction to go is unambiguous, the tree is shallow, but where the situation is ambiguous, the tree is deep. As a case in point, consider the hallways that have a code of 10. The decision for what direction to take next is very ambiguous but can be resolved with a local history of the agent's recent perceptions and actions. The figure shows that the tree accomplishes this

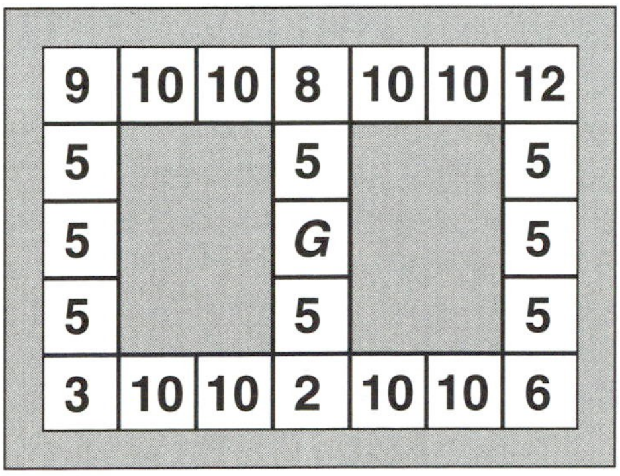

Figure 11.18 A hallway navigation task with limited sensors. World locations are labeled with integers that encode the four bits of perception. (From McCallum, 1995b. © MIT.)

Algorithm 11.4 Utile Distinction Memory

1. Initialize the history tree so that it is initially empty.

2. Make a move in the environment, and record the result in the instance chain.

3. Add the instance to the history tree.

4. Do one step of value iteration.

5. Test the fringe of the tree using the Kolmogorov-Smirnoff test.

6. Choose the next action such that

$$u_{t+1} = \text{argmax}\, Q[L(T_t), u]$$

or choose a random action and explore.

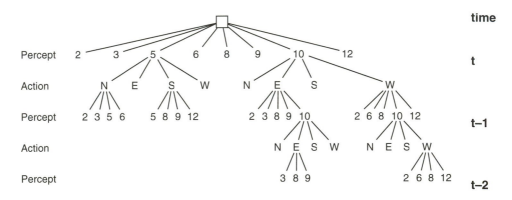

Figure 11.19 A tree for navigating through the environment in the maze task. Deeper branches of the tree correspond to longer, more detailed memories. Memory was created only where needed to solve the task at hand. (From McCallum, 1995b. © MIT.)

purpose. This algorithm is an instance of the use of *decision trees* in learning and is only representative of a larger set of learning algorithms that use such trees as a memory structure.[14] The main reason for its prominence here is its use of reinforcement learning.

11.8 SUMMARY

When exploring a state space of uncertain rewards, an agent can learn what to do by keeping track of its state history and appropriately propagating rewards. Initially we assumed that this exploration can be completely characterized; in other words, the world and the agent's model of that world are identical. The hard (and more interesting) part occurs when this assumption is not true, and the agent must decide what to do based on a description of the world that is necessarily incomplete. This incompleteness is a mixed blessing. It is a drawback when the agent needs to distinguish two world states but in fact does not. However, leverage may be gained by not distinguishing states for which the control policy is identical. The techniques for studying the aliased case must construct the state space based on a series of observations of its actions, observations, and rewards.

Critics of reinforcement learning as a model for the brain's programming are quick to point out the time-consuming nature of the algorithm, but there are ameliorating factors. First, once a model of the state space and actions has been learned, the time to find the solution is much faster, as dynamic programming can be used. Second, reinforcement learning, in principle, can use its model in simulation,[15] although this effort has so far only been made in very limited circumstances. The simulation would be entirely neural so that the results would be obtained much faster in this planning mode, wherein the rewards for bad results are just secondary rewards. Third, studies of human performance suggest that humans have many ways to keep the state space for any particular problem small.[16] A final point to make is that for most learning scenarios there is so far no good biological alternative to the secondary-reward mechanism as an explanation of how programming gets done.

NOTES

1. R. H. Canon, *Dynamics of Physical Systems* (New York: McGraw-Hill, 1967).

2. C. J. C. H. Watkins and P. Dayan, "Q-Learning," *Machine Learning* 8 (1992):279.

3. Developed by R. S. Sutton and A. G. Barto in "Time-Derivative Models of Pavlovian Reinforcement," in M. Gabriel and J. Moore, eds., *Learning and Computational Neuroscience: Foundations of Adaptive Networks* (Cambridge, MA: MIT Press, 1990).

4. P. Dayan, "The Convergence of TD(λ) for General λ," *Machine Learning* 8 (1992):341.

5. The figure is from Gerald Tesauro, "Practical Issues in Temporal Difference Learning," *Machine Learning* 8 (1992):257.

6. Steven D. Whitehead, "A Study of Cooperative Mechanisms for Faster Reinforcement Learning," Ph.D. thesis and TR 365, Computer Science Department, University of Rochester, February 1992.

7. Steven D. Whitehead and Dana H. Ballard, "Learning to Perceive and Act by Trial and Error," *Machine Learning* 7 (1991):45–83.

8. Due to Andrew Kachites McCallum, "Reinforcement Learning with Selective Perception and Hidden State," Ph.D. thesis, Computer Science Department, University of Rochester, December 1995b.

9. The idea of markers for this purpose was introduced by P. E. Agre and D. Chapman in "Pengi: An Implementation of a Theory of Activity," *Proceedings of the 6th National Conference on Artificial Intelligence* (AAAI-87) (Los Altos, CA: Morgan Kaufmann, 1987), pp. 268–72, building on work by Shimon Ullman described in "Visual Routines," *Cognition* 18 (1984): 97–157.

10. Lonnie Chrisman, "Reinforcement Learning with Perceptual Aliasing: The Perceptual Distinctions Approach," *Proceedings of the 10th National Conference on Artificial Intelligence* (AAAI-92) (Menlo Park, CA: AAAI Press, 1992), pp. 183–88.

11. McCallum, "Reinforcement Learning with Selective Perception and Hidden State."

12. R. Andrew McCallum, "Instance-Based State Identification for Reinforcement Learning," in G. Tesauro, D. Touretzky, and T. Leen, eds., *Advances in Neural Information Processing Systems,* vol. 7 (Cambridge, MA: MIT Press, 1995a).

13. McCallum, "Reinforcement Learning with Selective Perception and Hidden State."

14. See also B. D. Ripley, *Pattern Recognition and Neural Networks* (New York: Cambridge University Press, 1996); J. R. Quinlan and R. L. Rivest, "Inferring Decision Trees Using the Minimum Description Length Principle," *Information and Computation* 80 (1989):227–48; and J. R. Quinlan, "The Minimum Description Length Principle and Categorical Theories," in W. W. Cohen and H. Hirsh, eds., *Proceedings of the 11th International Machine Learning Conference* (San Francisco, CA: Morgan Kaufmann, 1994).

15. Richard S. Sutton, "First Results with DYNA, an Integrated Architecture for Learning, Planning, and Reacting," *Proceedings of the AAAI Spring Symposium on Planning in Uncertain, Unpredictable, or Changing Environments* (Menlo Park, CA: AAAI Press, 1990).

16. Dana H. Ballard, Mary M. Hayhoe, and Polly K. Pook, "Deictic Codes for the Embodiment of Cognition," *Behavioral and Brain Sciences,* in press.

EXERCISES

1. The network shown in Figure 11.20 represents a particular state of a network used by reinforcement learning. The numbers on each node are estimates of the value function, and the values for each of the actions, shown by arcs, are the current Q-values. Simulate by hand calculation one step of Q-learning for three of the nodes from the network with $\eta = \gamma = \frac{1}{2}$.

2. Why is reinforcement learning like dynamic programming?

3. In reinforcement learning, what is the role of the discount factor γ?

4. Implement a computer simulation of the pole-balancing problem. Plot the learning time as a function of the grain in the discretization space.

5. Use the pole-balancing example to test the LEC and LBW models.

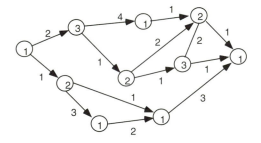

Figure 11.20   A network used by reinforcement learning. The values at each node n are $V(n)$, and the values on each action arc are the associated Q-values. The network is shown in an unconverged state.

IV   Systems

In the foregoing sections, learning algorithms can be seen as operating as if they had knowledge of a minimization principle termed minimum-description-length. But how do the algorithms "know" about this principle? Herein we introduce the final set of algorithms based on Darwin's theory of evolution. The astonishing feature is that the algorithms do not have to "know" about the principle at all! The right thing will happen as long as (1) variations of the algorithms can be produced in different animals of the species and (2) the environment can reward good algorithms with higher probabilities of survival. The nature of evolution's undirected directedness is very counterintuitive.[1,2]

GENE PRIMER

Let's start by looking at the biological setting. A species' population contains individuals, each with a set of *chromosomes*. Human chromosomes come in pairs. Each pair of chromosomes is a very long string of DNA containing *genes* at given loci, as shown in Figure IV.1.[3] The genes are also in pairs owing to their chromosomes. Pairs of genes are termed *alleles*. Each allele can represent a different trait or the same trait. Different traits are termed heterozygous; alike traits are termed homozygous. During sexual reproduction, the chromosome pairs from each sex split up into singletons (haploid) and then recombine (diploid). After this process the chromosome *genotype* is read by numerous proteins to construct an individual, termed a *phenotype*. Of the pairs of genes, only one, the *dominant gene*, is used in the building process; the unused gene is *recessive*. Thus we can see that there is a one-in-four chance that a particular gene from one of the sexual partners is dominant.

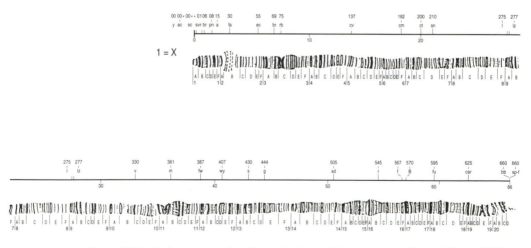

Figure IV.1 A chromosome is a linear structure with genes at specific loci. (From Wallace, 1992.)

Besides this basic splitting and pairing, there are other ways of modifying the new pairs:

- In *crossover*, subsequences of genes from the pairs may be exchanged.
- In *inversion*, a subsequence may appear in inverted order.
- In *mutation*, a single gene may be randomly changed.

In a vertebrate there are tens of thousands of genes, so that, assuming two alleles per gene, there are $2^{10,000} \approx 10^{3,000}$ different individuals that are possible. So in the present population of about 5 billion, only a tiny fraction of the number of possible individuals are represented.

The process of creating an individual or *phenotype* has many *epistatic* (nonlinear) effects. For one thing, the chemical building process depends on sequences of gene loci. For another, there are many additional environmental effects, such as competing species. Thus the fitness function that rates each genetic code is a highly nonlinear function of loci permutations. Nonetheless, despite these caveats, genes specify the building of components of living things and are very much the genesis for biological programs that build them. A stunning demonstration of this fact was the splicing of the gene related to building a mouse eye into the genetic code for a fly. The fly developed with a faceted eye at the end of its antennae (Figure IV.2), showing that the "code" for an eye was interpretable across this huge species gulf.[4]

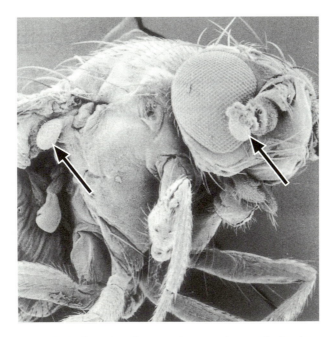

Figure IV.2 Scanning electron microscope image of a fly after gene transplant showing ectopic eyes under the wing and on the antennae (arrows). (From Halder, Callaerts, and Gehring, 1995; reprinted with permission from *Science*, © 1995 American Association for the Advancement of Science.)

Despite the huge number of genes, there are not enough to specify the 10^{14} synapses of the neurons in the brain, so the function of the genes has to be limited to more gross architectural features such as the wiring patterns.

LEARNING ACROSS GENERATIONS: SYSTEMS

Look-up tables and reinforcement strategies can reconfigure the existing structures, but to alter the hardware design, genetic changes are needed. Modeling the genetic process dates from the work of Holland in the 1960s.[5] Such *genetic algorithms* model the alteration of the genes during reproduction in order to create new architectural forms. These algorithms can be understood as experimenting with brain hardware and the structure of the body. The brain occupies the position of central importance: It is believed that about one-third of the DNA is used to design the brain. The gross features of the brain are relatively similar across mammals. For example, humans and chimps seem to have about 98% of their DNA in common. However, there are dramatic differences in certain details. For example, in cats the connections from the LGN enervate many disparate visual cortical areas, but in humans and monkeys, the connections are limited to cortical visual area V1. Such differences in turn affect the choice of software that gets learned.

Changing hardware is a slow process that operates across millions of generations; nevertheless, genetic algorithms are comparable in power to algorithms derived from developmental and behavioral learning.

The process of decoding DNA to construct amino acids, complicated proteins, and ultimately the exquisite structures that are living forms is incredibly complex. Genetic algorithms are huge abstractions that capture just the overall features of the reproductive process.

• They use a coding of the problem to be solved in a DNA-like string.

• The search uses a substantial population of state space points rather than a single point.

• The control of the population is governed by a *fitness function* that rates each individual.

• The reproductive rules are nondeterministic.

Since genetic algorithm (GA) search uses a population and nondeterministic reproductive rules, one might think that the secret to its success is just random search. However, it has been shown that GA populations are vastly more efficient than just guessing new state space points. As the parameters governing the search have become better understood, there have been remarkable successes. For example, a GA has produced a program that replicates itself and that is shorter than those designed by human programmers.[6] The force behind the genetic algorithm is captured in the *schemata theorem*. This shows that if any piece of the DNA confers an above-average survival rate on its host, then there is a good chance that that piece will spread through the population at an exponential rate. Thus sexual reproduction promotes the rapid spread of good algorithmic features. Its various DNA-shuffling mechanisms also provide a way of trying out new features. Remarkably, our brains owe their existence to this "blind watchmaking" process.[7]

There are two main types of genetic algorithms: standard GAs and the more recently developed *genetic programming*.[8]

Standard Genetic Algorithms

Genetic algorithms use strings of symbols to represent the genetic code and a fitness function to score the code. Populations of strings represent a species, and the most fit species represents the best solution found so far. The operations of sexual combination are translated into operations on the symbol strings, so that the population of symbol strings can evolve through "sexual" reproduction. Search proceeds by preferentially selecting the fittest strings for reproduction.

Genetic Programming

Biologically, DNA is only part of the story. Proteins must be manufactured, which in turn assemble the phenotype, or living individual. In standard GAs all this is implicitly incorporated into the fitness function. This function scores the entire process, although it is never explicitly represented. In contrast, genetic programs represent individuals as actual programs. The genetic operations are carried out on the program code. That is, the string representing the "DNA" is also representing an individual as a functioning program. As a consequence, the program can be directly tested in an environment of data. Therefore, the fitness function has less to do. Adding the additional structure of a program operating on data also allows the encoding of the problem to be more refined, in turn leading to better fitness functions. At this time, picking good fitness functions is very much an art form, although there has been very recent work in describing hierarchical fitness functions.

NOTES

1. Richard Dawkins, *The Selfish Gene* (New York: Oxford University Press, 1989).

2. Daniel C. Dennett, *Darwin's Dangerous Idea: Evolution and the Meanings of Life* (New York: Simon and Schuster, 1995).

3. Bruce Wallace, *The Search for the Gene* (Ithaca, NY: Cornell University Press, 1992), p. 72.

4. Georg Halder, Patrick Callaerts, and Walter J. Gehring, "Induction of Ectopic Eyes by Targeted Expression of Eyeless Gene in *Drosophila*," *Science* 267 (March 1995):1788–92.

5. John H. Holland, *Adaptation in Natural and Artificial Systems: An Introductory Analysis with Applications to Biology, Control, and Artificial Intelligence*, 2nd ed. (1st ed., 1975) (Cambridge, MA: MIT Press, Bradford, 1992).

6. Thomas S. Ray, "Evolution, Complexity, Entropy, and Artificial Reality," *Physica D* 75, no. 1/3 (August 1, 1994):239.

7. Richard Dawkins, *The Blind Watchmaker* (New York: Norton, 1986).

8. John R. Koza, *Genetic Programming: On the Programming of Computers by Means of Natural Selection* (Cambridge, MA: MIT Press, Bradford, 1992).

12 Genetic Algorithms

ABSTRACT   Genetic algorithms (GA) is an optimization technique for searching very large spaces that models the role of the genetic material in living organisms. A small population of individual exemplars can effectively search a large space because they contain *schemata,* useful substructures that can be potentially combined to make fitter individuals. Formal studies of competing schemata show that the best policy for replicating them is to increase them exponentially according to their relative fitness. This turns out to be the policy used by genetic algorithms. Fitness is determined by examining a large number of individual fitness cases. This process can be very efficient if the fitness cases also evolve by their own GAs.

12.1   INTRODUCTION

Network models, such as multilayered perceptrons, make local changes and so find local minima. To find more global minima a different kind of algorithm is called for. Genetic algorithms fill the bill. These algorithms also allow large changes in the state to be made easily. They have a number of distinct properties:

• They work with an encoding of the parameters.

• They search by means of a population of individuals.

• They use a *fitness function* that does not require the calculation of derivatives.

• They search probabilistically.

   In broad outline the idea of a GA is to encode the problem in a string. For example, if the problem is to find the maximum of a scalar function $f(x)$, the string can be obtained by representing x in binary. A population represents a diverse set of strings that are different possible solutions to the problem. The fitness function scores each of these as to its optimality. In the example, the associated value of f for each binary string is its fitness. At each generation, operators produce new individuals (strings) that are on average fitter. After a given set of generations, the fittest member in the population is chosen as the answer.

   The two key parameters are the number of generations N_G and the population size N_p. If the population is too small, there will not be sufficient diversity in the strings to find the optimal string by a series of operations. If the number of generations is too small, there will not be enough chances to find the optimum. These two parameters are not independent. The larger the population, the smaller the number of generations needed to have a good chance of finding the optimum. Note that the optimum is not guaranteed; there is just a good chance of finding it. Certain problems will be very hard (technically they are called *deceptive* if the global minimum is hard to find). Note that for the solution to be not found, the probability of generating it from the population as it traverses the generations has to be small.

The structure of a GA uses a reproductive plan that works as shown in Algorithm 12.1.

The raw fitness score for the *i*th individual, $h(i)$, is any way of assessing good solutions that you have. Of course the performance of the algorithm will be sensitive to the function that you pick. Rather than work with h, it is more useful to convert raw fitness to normalized fitness f, where

$$f(i) = \frac{h(i)}{\sum_{i=1}^{N_p} h(i)}$$

Since now $\sum_{i=1}^{N_p} f(i) = 1$, this method allows the fitness values to be used as probabilities.

Probabilistic operations enter the algorithm in three different phases. First, the initial population must be selected. This choice can be made randomly (or if you have some special knowledge of good starting points, these can be chosen). Next, members of the population have to be selected for reproduction. One way is to select individuals based on fitness, produce offspring, score the offspring, and then delete individuals from the resultant population based on $1 - f$. The third way probabilities enter into consideration is in the selection of the genetic operation to be used.

Algorithm 12.1   The Genetic Algorithm

Choose a population size.

Choose the number of generations N_G.

Initialize the population.

Repeat the following for N_G generations:

1. Select a given number of pairs of individuals from the population probabilistically after assigning each structure a probability proportional to observed performance.

2. Copy the selected individual(s), then apply *operators* to them to produce new individual(s).

3. Select other individuals at random and replace them with the new individuals.

4. Observe and record the fitness of the new individuals.

Output the fittest individual as the answer.

12.1.1 Genetic Operators

Now let's define the genetic operators. Let the symbol a denote a gene, and denote a chromosome by a sequence of genes $a_1a_2a_3\ldots a_n$. The set of alleles $c_{i1},\ldots,c_{ij_i}$ represents the possible codes that can be used at location i. Thus the gene will represent one of these

$$a_i \in c_{i1},\ldots,c_{ij_i}$$

but to take a specific example, for an alphabet of the first three letters, the alleles would be $\{a, b, c\}$ at every position.

The first operator is *crossover,* wherein subsequences of two parent strings are interchanged. The point of the operator is to combine two good subsequences on the same string. To implement the operation, crossover points must be selected probabilistically. Then the substrings are swapped, as shown in Figure 12.1 (*top*).

Once good subsequences appear in an individual, it is advantageous to preserve them from being broken up by further crossover operations. Shorter subsequences have a better chance of surviving crossover. For that reason the *inversion* operation is useful for moving good sequences closer together. Inversion is defined in the middle section of Figure 12.1.

As the GA progresses, the diversity of the population may be removed as the individuals all take on the characteristics of an exemplar from a local minimum. In this case *mutation* is a way to introduce diversity into the population and avoid local minima. Mutation works by choosing an element of the string at random and replacing it with another symbol from the code, as shown in the bottom section of Figure 12.1.

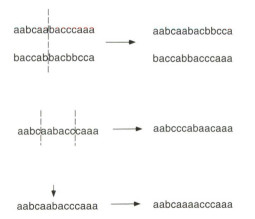

Figure 12.1 Genetic operations on a three-letter alphabet of $\{a, b, c\}$. (*top*) Crossover swaps strings at a crossover point. (*middle*) Inversion reverses the order of letters in a substring. (*bottom*) Mutation changes a single element.

12.1.2 An Example

Consider finding the maximum of the function $f(x) = -x^2 + 12x + 300$ where x takes on integer values $0, \dots, 31$. This example is easily solved with direct methods, but it will be encoded as a GA search problem to demonstrate the operations involved.

The first step in defining the GA is to code the search space. The encoding used for genetic operations is the binary code for the independent variable x. The value of $f(x)$ is the fitness value. Normalized fitness over the whole population determines the probability P_{select} of being selected for reproduction. Table 12.1 shows an initial condition for the algorithm starting with five individuals.

Now select two individuals for reproduction. Selections are made by accessing a random number generator, using the probabilities shown in the column P_{select}. Suppose that individuals 2 and 4 are picked.

The operation we will use is crossover, which requires picking a locus on the string for the crossover site. This is also done using a random number generator. Suppose the result is two, counting the front as zero. The two new individuals that result are shown in Table 12.2 along with their fitness values. Now these new individuals have to be added to the population, maintaining population size. Thus it is necessary to select individuals for removal. Once again the random number generator is consulted. Suppose that individuals 1 and 3 lose this contest. The result of one iteration of the GA is shown in Table 12.3.

Note that after this operation the average fitness of the population has increased. You might be wondering why the best individuals are not selected at the expense of the worst. Why go to the trouble of using the fitness values? The reason can be appreciated by considering what would happen if it turned out that all the best individuals had their last bit set to 1.

Table 12.1   Initial condition for the genetic algorithm example.

Individual	Genetic Code	x	$f(x)$	P_{select}
1	10110	22	80	0.08
2	10001	17	215	0.22
3	11000	24	12	0.01
4	00010	2	320	0.33
5	00111	7	335	0.36
Average			192	

Table 12.2   Mating process.

Mating Pair	Site	New Individual	$f(x)$	P_{select}
00010	2	10010	192	0.14
10001	2	00001	311	0.23

Table 12.3 The genetic algorithm example after one step.

Individual	Genetic Code	x	$f(x)$	P_{select}
1	10010	18	192	0.14
2	10001	17	215	0.16
3	00001	1	311	0.23
4	00010	2	320	0.23
5	00111	7	335	0.24
Average			275	

There would be no way to fix this situation by crossover. The solution has a 0 in the last bit position, and there would be no way to generate such an individual. In this case the small population would get stuck at a local minimum. Now you see why the low-fitness individuals are kept around: they are a source of diversity with which to cover the solution space.

12.2 SCHEMATA

In very simple form, the example exhibits an essential property of the genetic coding: that individual loci in the code can confer fitness on the individual. Since the optimum is 6, all individuals with their leading bit set to 0 will be fit, regardless of the rest of the bits. In general, the extent to which loci can confer independent fitness will simplify the search. If the bits were completely independent, they could be tested individually and the problem would be very simple, so the difficulty of the problem is related to the extent to which the bits interact in the fitness calculation.

A way of getting a handle on the impact of sets of loci is the concept of *schemata* (singular: schema).[1] A schema denotes a subset of strings that have identical values at certain loci. The form of a schema is a template in which the common bits are indicated explicitly and a "don't care" symbol (*) is used to indicate the irrelevant part of the string (from the standpoint of the schema). For example, 1 * 101 denotes the strings {10101, 11101}. Schemata contain information about the diversity of the population. For example, a population of n individuals using a binary genetic code of length l contains somewhere between 2^l and $n2^l$ schemata.

Not all schemata are created equal, because of the genetic operations, which tend to break up some schemata more than others. For example, 1 * * * * 1 is more vulnerable to crossover than * 11 * * *. In general, short schemata will be the most robust.

12.2.1 Schemata Theorem

To see the importance of schemata, let's track the number of representatives of a given schema in a population. It turns out that the growth of a particular schema in a population is very easy to determine. Let t be a variable that denotes a particular generation, and let $m(S, t)$ be the number of schema exemplars in a population at generation t. To simplify matters, ignore the effects of crossover in breaking up schema. Then the number of this schema in the new population is directly proportional to the chance of an individual being picked that has the schema. Considering the entire population, this is

$$m(S, t + 1) = m(S, t)n\frac{f(S)}{\sum_i f_i}$$

because an individual is picked with probability $\frac{f(S)}{\sum_i f_i}$ and there are n picks. This equation can be written more succinctly as

$$m(S, t + 1) = m(S, t)\frac{f(S)}{f_{ave}}$$

To see the effects of this equation more vividly, adopt the further simplifying assumption that $f(S)$ remains above the average fitness by a constant amount. That is, for some c, write

$$f(S) = f_{ave}(1 + c)$$

Then it is easy to show that

$$m(S, t) = m(S, 0)(1 + c)^t$$

In other words, for a fitness that is slightly above the mean, the number of schema instances will grow exponentially, whereas if the fitness is slightly below the average (c negative), the schema will decrease exponentially. This equation is just an approximation because it ignores things like new schemata that can be created with the operators, but nonetheless it captures the main dynamics of schema growth.

12.2.2 The Bandit Problem

The upshot of the previous analysis has been to show that fit schemata propagate exponentially at a rate that is proportional to their relative fitness. Why is this a good thing to do? The answer can be developed in terms of a related problem, the two-armed bandit problem (Las Vegas slot machines are nicknamed "one-armed bandits"). The two-armed slot machine is constructed so that the arms have different payoffs. The problem for the gambler is to pick the arm with the higher payoff. If the arms had the same payoff on each pull the problem would be easy. Just pull each lever once and then pull the winner after that. The problem is that the arms pay a random amount, say with means m_1 and m_2 and corresponding variances σ_1 and σ_2.

This problem can be analyzed by choosing a fixed strategy for N trials. One such strategy is to pull both levers n times (where $2n < N$) and then pull the best for the remaining number of trials. The expected loss for this strategy is

$$L(N, n) = |m_1 - m_2| \{(N - n)p(n) + n[1 - p(n)]\} \qquad (12.1)$$

where $p(n)$ is the probability that the arm that is actually worst looks the best after n trials. We can approximate $p(n)$ by

$$p(n) \approx \frac{e^{-x^2/2}}{\sqrt{2\pi x}}$$

where

$$x = \frac{m_1 - m_2}{\sqrt{\sigma_1^2 + \sigma_2^2}} \sqrt{n}$$

With quite a bit of work this equation can be differentiated with respect to n to find the optimal experiment size n^*. The net result is that the total number of trials grows at a rate that is greater than an exponential function of n^*. More refined analyses can be done, but they only confirm the basic result: Once you think you know the best lever, you should pull that lever an exponentially greater number of times. You only keep pulling the bad lever on the remote chance that you are wrong. This result generalizes to the k-armed bandit problem. Resources should be allocated among the k arms so that the best arms receive an exponentially increasing number of trials, in proportion to their estimated advantage.

In the light of this result, let us return to the analysis of schemata. In particular, consider schemata that compete with each other. For example, the following schemata all compete with each other:

$$* * 0 * 0 0 *$$
$$* * 0 * 0 1 *$$
$$* * 0 * 1 0 *$$
$$* * 0 * 1 1 *$$
$$* * 1 * 0 0 *$$
$$* * 1 * 0 1 *$$
$$* * 1 * 1 0 *$$
$$* * 1 * 1 1 *$$

Do you see the relationship between the bandit problem and schema? If these schemata act independently to confer fitness on the individuals that contain them, then the number of each schema should be increased exponentially according to its relative fitness. But this is what the GA is doing!

Summary   You should recognize that all of the foregoing discussion has not been a proof that GAs work, but merely an argument. The summary of the argument is as follows:

• GAs seem to work. In practice, they find solutions much faster (with higher probability) than would be expected from random search.

• If all the bits in the GA encoding were independent, it would be a simple matter to optimize over each one of the bits independently. This is not the case, but the belief is that for many problems, one can optimize over sub-sets of bits. In GAs these are schemata.

• Short schemata have a high probability of surviving the genetic operations.

• Focusing on short schemata that compete shows that, over the short run, the fittest are increasing at an exponential rate.

• This has been shown to be the right thing to do for the bandit problem, which optimizes reward for competing alternatives with probabilistic pay-offs that have stable statistics.

• Ergo, if all of the assumptions hold (we cannot tell whether they do, but we suspect they do), GAs are optimal.

12.3   DETERMINING FITNESS

In the simple example used to illustrate the basic mechanisms of the GA, fitness could be calculated directly from the code. In general, though, it may depend on a number of *fitness cases* taken from the environment. For example, suppose the problem is to find a parity function over binary in-puts of length four. All 2^4 inputs may have to be tested on each individual in the population. In these kinds of problems, fitness is often usefully de-fined as the fraction of successful answers to the fitness cases. When the number of possible cases is small, they can be exhaustively tested, but as this number becomes large, the expense of the overall algorithm increases proportionately. This is the impetus for some kind of approximation method that would reduce the cost of the fitness calculation. The following sections describe two methods for controlling this cost.

12.3.1   Racing for Fitness

One of the simplest ways of economizing on the computation of fitness is to estimate fitness from a limited sample. Suppose that the fitness score is the mean of the fitnesses for each of the samples, or fitness cases. As these are evaluated, the estimate of the mean becomes more and more accurate. The fitness estimate is going to be used for the selection of members of the population for reproduction. It may well be that this fitness can be esti-mated to a useful level of accuracy long before the entire retinue of fitness cases has been evaluated.[2] The estimate of fitness is simply the average of the individual fitness cases tested so far. Assuming there are n of them, the sample mean is given by

$$\bar{f} = \frac{1}{n} \sum_{i=1}^{n} f_i$$

and the sample variance by

$$s^2 = \frac{1}{n-1} \sum_{i=1}^{n} (f_i - \bar{f})^2$$

Given that many independent estimates are being summed, make the assumption that the distribution of estimates of fitness is normal, that is, $N(\mu, \sigma)$. Then the marginal posterior distribution of the mean is a Student distribution with mean $\bar{f}$, variance s/n, and $n - 1$ degrees of freedom. A Student distribution is the distribution of the random variable $t = \frac{(\bar{f} - \mu)\sqrt{n-1}}{s}$, which is a way of estimating the mean of a normal distribution that does not depend on the variance.[3] The cumulative density function can be used to design a test for acceptance of the estimate. Once the sample mean is sufficiently close to the mean, testing fitness cases can be discontinued, and the estimate can be used in the reproduction phase.

Example: Testing Two Fitness Cases Suppose that we have the sample means and variances of the fitness cases for two different individuals after ten tests. These are $\bar{f}_1 = 21, \bar{f}_2 = 17$, and $s_1 = 3$. Let us stop testing if the two means are significantly different at the 5% level. To do so, choose an interval $(-a, a)$ such that

$P(-a < t < a) = 0.95$

Since $n - 1 = 9$, there are 9 degrees of freedom. A table for the Student distribution with nine degrees of freedom shows that

$P(-2.26 < t < 2.26) = 0.95$

Now for the test use the sample mean of the second distribution as the hypothetical mean of the first; that is,

$$t = \frac{(\bar{f}_1 - \bar{f}_2)\sqrt{n-1}}{s_1}$$

With $\bar{f}_1 = 21, \bar{f}_2 = 17$, and $s_1 = 3$,

$t = 4$

which is outside of the range of 95% probability. Thus we can conclude that the means are significantly different and stop the test.

12.3.2   Coevolution of Parasites

Up to this point the modeling effort has focused on a single species. But we know that "nature is red in tooth and claw"; that is, the competition between different species can improve the fitness on each. To demonstrate this principle we will study the example of efficient sorting networks. This example was introduced by Hillis,[4] who also introduced new features to the basic genetic algorithm.

The idea of a sorting network is shown in Figure 12.2. Numbers appear at the input lines on the left. At each crossbar joining two lines, the numbers are compared and then swapped if the higher number is on the lower line (and otherwise left unchanged).

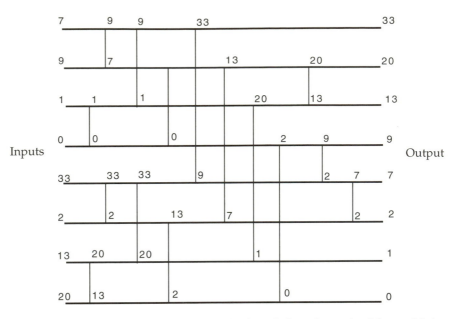

Figure 12.2 An eight-element sorting network. The eight lines denote the eight possible inputs. A vertical bar between the lines means that the values on those lines are swapped at that point. The disposition of the particular input sample is tracked through the network by showing the results of the swaps.

Recalling the basic result from complexity analysis that sorting takes at least $n \log n$ operations, you might think that the best 16-input network would contain at least 64 swaps.[5] This result holds in the limit of large n. For small 16-input networks, a solution has been found that does the job in 60 swaps. Hillis shows that a GA encoding can find a 65-swap network, but that introducing parasites results in a 61-swap network.

The encoding for the sorting problem distinguishes a model genotype from a phenotype. In the genotype a chromosome is a sequence of pairs of numbers. Each pair specifies the lines that are to be tested for swapping at that point in the network. A diploid encoding contains a second chromosome with a similar encoding.

To create a phenotype, the chromosome pair is used as follows. At each gene location, if the alleles are the same—that is, have the same pairs of numbers—then only one pair is used. If they are different, then both are used (see Figure 12.3). The result is that heterozygous pairs result in larger sorting networks, whereas homozygous pairs result in shorter networks. The advantage of this encoding strategy is that the size of the network does not have to be explicitly included in the fitness function. If a sequence is useful, it is likely to appear in many genes and will thus automatically shorten the network during the creation of the phenotype.

The fitness function is the percentage of the sequences that are sorted correctly. Experience shows that indexing the mating program with spatial locality is helpful. Rather than randomly selecting mates solely on fitness,

Chapter 12 Genetic Algorithms

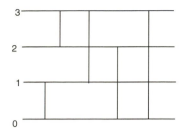

(0 1)(2 3)(1 3)(0 2)
(0 1)(2 3)(1 3)(0 3)

Figure 12.3 The translation of genotype to phenotype used by Hillis demonstrated on a four-input sorting network. The genetic code contains a haploid representation with two possible swaps at each location. When the possible swaps are identical, only one is used in constructing the phenotype, resulting in a shorter network. In the example, the last pair results in two links, the second of which is redundant.

each individual is assigned a location on a two-dimensional grid. The choice of mates is biased according to a Gaussian distribution, which is a function of grid distance.

Another nice property of the sorting networks is that just testing them with sequences of 0s and 1s is sufficient; if the network works for all permutations of 0s and 1s, it will work for any sequence of numbers.[6] Even so, it is still prohibitively expensive to use all 2^{16} test cases of 0s and 1s to evaluate fitness. Instead, a subset of cases is used. A problem with this approach is that the resultant networks tend to cluster around solutions that get most of the cases right but cannot handle a few difficult examples. This limitation is the motivation for parasites. Parasites represent sets of test cases. They evolve similarly, breeding by combining the test cases that they represent. They are rewarded for the reverse of the networks: the number of cases that the network gets wrong. The parasites keep the sorting-network population from getting stuck in a local minimum. If that outcome occurs, then the parasites will evolve test cases targeted expressly at this population. A further advantage of parasites is that testing is more efficient.

NOTES

1. The exposition here follows David E. Goldberg's text *Genetic Algorithms in Search, Optimization, and Machine Learning* (Reading, MA: Addison-Wesley, 1989), which has much additional detail.

2. This idea has been proposed by A. W. Moore and M. S. Lee in "Efficient Algorithms for Minimizing Cross Validation Error," *Proceedings of the 11th International Machine Learning Conference* (San Mateo, CA: Morgan Kaufmann, 1994). In their proposal they advocate using gradient search instead of the full-blown mechanics of a genetic algorithm, and show that it

works well for simple problems. Of course, since gradient search is a local algorithm, its over-all effectiveness will be a function of the structure of the search space.

3. H. D. Brunk, *An Introduction to Mathematical Statistics,* 3rd ed. (Lexington, MA: Xerox College, 1975).

4. Daniel W. Hillis, "Co-evolving Parasites Improve Simulated Evolution as an Optimization Procedure," in Christopher Langton et al., eds., *Artificial Life II,* SFI Studies in the Sciences of Complexity, vol. 10 (Reading, MA: Addison-Wesley, 1991).

5. Thomas H. Cormen, Charles E. Leiserson, and Ronald L. Rivest, *Introduction to Algorithms* (Cambridge, MA: MIT Press, 1990).

6. Ibid.

EXERCISES

1. Use a GA encoding to find the maximum of

$$-2x^2 + 28x + 50$$

Plot the course of your population over time.

2. Suppose fitness in a binary string is measured as the number of 1s. Find the average fitness of a population of size N containing individuals of length k bits.

3. Design a GA to solve the traveling salesman problem. Which operators would work, and which would have problems? Test your algorithm on easy and hard data sets.

4. Differentiate the expression for loss $L(N, n)$ (Equation 12.1) to show that the optimal strategy is to pull the better lever more than an exponential number of times more frequently than the worse lever.

5. Modify the predator-prey model of Chapter 5 to allow the population of predators and prey to become fitter. How does this affect the stability of the population?

6. The ability to learn over a lifetime can improve fitness, as shown by G. E. Hinton and S. J. Nowlan, "How Learning Can Guide Evolution," *Complex Systems* 1 (1987):495–502. Suppose an individual has a 20-bit code, and that evolution is allowed to pick 10 of the bits. Survival requires that all 20 bits be set correctly. During its lifetime, the phenotype tries to find the correct settings for the unspecified bits by guessing them. Its fitness is measured in terms of the number of trials needed to find the correct solution:

$$f = 1 + \frac{19n}{1000}$$

Simulate this experiment with a population size of 250 to show the fundamental effect that even though the bits in the solutions found by the phenotypes are not *inherited* by their offspring, the experience of learning can help choose individuals whose inherited bits are part of the solution.

7. In the problem of the prisoners' dilemma, two prisoners can get 2-year sentences by not testifying against each other. However, if one of them

does testify against the other, he or she gets off free and the other gets a stiff 5-year sentence. The prisoners are not allowed to communicate beforehand. In the more interesting *iterated* prisoners' dilemma, the participants observe each other's strategy and form their own as a consequence. One GA encoding of this problem takes into account the most recent history. Where the participants either cooperate (C) or not (N), a partial strategy for just the most recent history would look like the following:

```
if CC then C
```

meaning "If I cooperated last time, and so did my collaborator, then I'll also cooperate next time." All four cases need to be represented. The purpose of the GA should be to pick the decision that maximizes payoff.

Try this for longer strategies, such as basing the decision on the last three interactions, that is,

```
if CC CC CC then C
```

using two versions of the GA to interact with each other.

13   Genetic Programming

ABSTRACT   Genetic programming (GP) applies the genetic algorithm directly to programs. The generality of programs allows many different problems to be tackled with the same methodology. Experimental results show that even though GP is searching a vast space, it has a high probability of generating successful results. Extensions to the basic GP algorithm add subroutines as primitives. This has been shown to greatly increase the efficiency of the search.

13.1   INTRODUCTION

In genetic algorithms the problem is encoded as a string. This means that there is always a level of indirection whereby the meaning of the string has to be interpreted. A more direct way of solving a problem would be to have the string encode the *program* for solving the problem. Then the search strategy would be to have the genetic operations act on the programs themselves. The advantage of this approach would be that programs could rate themselves according to how well they are doing and rewrite themselves to do better. The difficulty is that, in general, making a change to a program will be disastrous to its function. To make it work, there must be some way of encoding changes that makes the genetic modifications less destructive. This is the goal of *genetic programming,* which works directly with programs encoded as trees instead of strings.

A beautiful idea is to use the LISP programming language.[1] This is a functional language based on lists. For example, the function called $f(x, y)$ is encoded simply as

```
(f x y)
```

which is a function followed by a list of arguments to that function. Running the program, or *evaluating the function,* results in the value of the function being computed. For example, evaluating the LISP list

```
(* 3 4)
```

results in a value of 12. Complex programs are expressed by using composite functions. For example,

```
(+ 2 (IF (> X 3) 4 7))
```

evaluates to 6 if X is greater than 3; otherwise it evaluates to 9. The list structure consists of *terminals* and *functions*. For instance, in the present example,

```
{x,2,3,4,7}
```

are terminals, whereas

```
{IF, +, >}
```

are functions.[2]

Every LISP program has this simple list structure. This has several advantages:

• The uniform list structure represents both program code and data. This simple syntax allows genetic operations to be simply defined.

• The format of the instructions is one of a function applied to arguments. This represents the control information in a common syntax, which is again amenable to modification with genetic operators.

• The variable-length structure of lists escapes the fixed-length limitation of the strings used in genetic algorithms.

13.2   GENETIC OPERATORS FOR PROGRAMS

A LISP program can be written as a nested list and drawn as a tree. The former fact is helpful because it allows the definition of the effects of operators on programs. The latter fact helps immensely because it allows the straightforward visualization of these effects. For example,

```
(* x (+ x y))
```

and

```
(+ (* z y) (/ y x))
```

can be thought of as representing the programs that compute $x(x + y)$ and $zy + y/x$. These programs in their list structure can be interpreted also as trees, as in Figure 13.1.

Operators have a very elegant structure in the list format. The first step in applying an operator consists of identifying *fracture points* in the list for

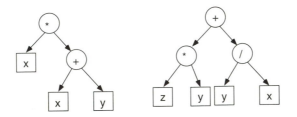

Figure 13.1   Functions in LISP can be interpreted as trees. Two examples are $(* x (+ x y))$ and $(+ (* z y)(/ y x))$.

Chapter 13   Genetic Programming

modification. These are analogous to crossover points in the string representation used by genetic algorithms. A fracture point may be either the beginning of a sublist or a terminal. The following examples illustrate the use of genetic operators.

To implement crossover, pick two individual programs. Next select any two sublists, one from each parent. Switch these sublists in the offspring. For example, pick y and (/ y x) from the two preceding examples. Then the offspring will be (* x (+ x (/ y x))) and (+ (* z y) y), shown in tree form in Figure 13.2.

To implement inversion, pick one individual from the population. Next select two fracture points within the individual. The new individual is obtained by switching the delimited subtrees. For example, using (+ (* z y) (/ y x)), let's pick z and (/ y x). The result is (+ (* (/ y x) y) z), shown in tree form in Figure 13.3.

To implement mutation, select one parent. Then replace randomly any function symbol with another function symbol or any terminal symbol with another terminal symbol. That is, (+ (* z y)(/ y x)) could become (+ (+ z y)(/ y x)), shown in tree form in Figure 13.4. Mutation may also be implemented by replacing a subtree with a new, randomly generated subtree.

What you have seen is that the genetic operators all have a very simple implementation in the LISP language owing to its list structure. But there is one caveat. These examples are all arithmetic functions that return integers, so there is no problem with swapping their arguments. However, there may be a problem if the results returned by the swapped functions are not commensurate. For example, if one function returns a list and it is

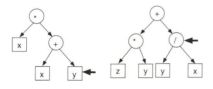

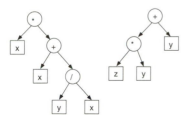

Figure 13.2   The genetic programming crossover operator works by picking fracture points in each of two programs. Then these sublists are swapped to produce two new offspring.

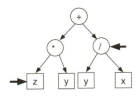

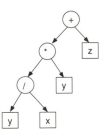

Figure 13.3 The genetic programming inversion operator works by picking two fracture points in a single program. These sublists are swapped to produce the new offspring.

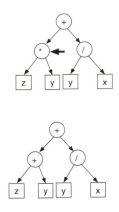

Figure 13.4 The genetic programming mutation operator works by picking a fracture point in a single program. Then the delimited terminal or nonterminal is changed to produce the new offspring.

swapped with another that returns an integer, the result will be a syntactically invalid structure. To avoid this error (at some cost), either all functions should return the same type of result, or some type of checking has to be implemented.

13.3 GENETIC PROGRAMMING

The structure of the genetic programming algorithm, Algorithm 13.1, is identical to that of the basic genetic algorithm (Algorithm 12.1). The principal difference is the interpretation of the string as a program. This difference shows up in the evaluation of fitness, wherein the program is tested on a set of inputs by evaluating it.

As examples of genetic programming we consider two problems. One is the parity problem: Given a set of binary inputs of fixed size n the program must correctly determine their parity. Although it is easy to build a parity function without using GP, this problem is valuable as a test case as it is a difficult problem for learning algorithms. Knowing the parity of subsets of the input is insufficient to predict the answer.

The second example is that of the Pac-Man video game. In this case the program must learn to control a robotic agent in a simulated environment that has rewards and punishments.

Example 1: Parity   Consider the problem of discovering the even-n parity function. The even-3 parity function is shown in Table 13.1. For this problem the terminals are given by three symbols that represent the three possible inputs to be tested for parity:

$T = \{D_0, D_1, D_2\}$

The function set is given by the set of primitive Boolean functions of two arguments

$F = \{AND, OR, NAND, NOR\}$

Using a population size of 4,000, a solution was discovered at generation 5. The solution contains 45 elements (the number of terminals plus the number of nonterminals). The individual comprising the solution is shown in the following program. As you can see, this solution is not the minimal function that could be written by hand but contains many uses of the

Algorithm 13.1   Genetic Programming

Choose a population size N_p.

Choose the number of generations N_G.

Initialize the population.

Repeat the following for N_G generations:

1. Select a given number of pairs of individuals from the population probabilistically after assigning each structure a probability proportional to observed performance.

2. Copy the selected structure(s), then apply *operators* to them to produce new structure(s).

3. Select other elements at random and replace them with the new structure(s).

4. Observe and record the fitness of the new structure.

Output the fittest individual as the answer.

Table 13.1 The even-3 parity function.

Input	Output
000	1
001	0
010	0
011	1
100	0
101	1
110	1
111	0

primitive function set, mostly because there is no pressure on the selection mechanism to choose minimal functions.

```
(AND (OR (OR D0 (NOR D1 D2)) D2)
     (AND (NAND (NOR (NOR D0 D2)
                     (AND (AND D1 D1) D1))
                (NAND (OR (AND D0 D1) D2) D0))
(OR (NAND (AND (D0 D2)
               (OR (NOR D0 (OR D2 D0) D1))
     (NAND (NAND D1 (NAND D0 D1)) D2)))
```

Example 2: Pac-Man   As another illustration of the use of GP, consider learning to play the game of Pac-Man.[3] The game is played on a 31×28 grid, as shown in Figure 13.5. At every time step, the Pac-Man can remain stationary or move one step in any possible direction in the maze. The goal of the game is to maximize points. Points are given for eating the food pellets arrayed along the maze corridors. Energizers are special objects and are worth 50 points each. At fixed times $t = 25$ and $t = 125$ a very valuable piece of fruit worth 2,000 points appears, moves on the screen for 75 time steps, and then disappears.

In the central den are four monsters. After the game begins they emerge from the den and chase the Pac-Man. If they catch him the game ends. Thus the game ends when the Pac-Man is eaten or when there is nothing left for him to eat. In this eat-or-be-eaten scenario the energizers play a valuable role. After the Pac-Man has eaten an energizer, all the monsters are vulnerable for 40 time steps and can be eaten. (In the video game the monsters turn blue for this period.) Thus a strategy for a human player is to lure the monsters close to an energizer, eat the energizer, and then eat the monster. Eating more than one monster is especially valuable. The first is worth 200 points, the next 400, the next 800, and the last 1600.

The monsters are as fast as the Pac-Man but are not quite as dogged. Of every 25 time steps, 20 are spent in pursuit of the Pac-Man and 5 in moving

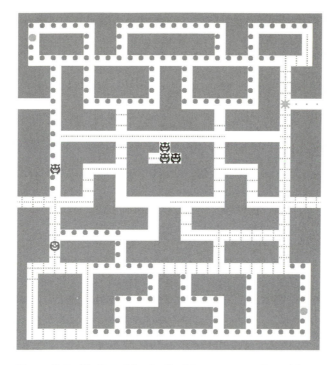

Figure 13.5 The board for the Pac-Man game, together with an example trace of a program found by genetic programming. The path of the Pac-Man is shown with vertical dots, and the paths of the monsters are shown with horizontal dots. In this example the Pac-Man starts in the middle of the second row from the bottom. The four monsters start in the central den. The Pac-Man first moves toward the upper right, where it captures a fruit and a pill, and subsequently attracts the monsters in the lower left corner. After eating a pill there it eats three monsters and almost catches the fourth. (From Rosca and Ballard, 1996.)

at random. But since there are more of them, they can succeed by cornering the Pac-Man.

The parity problem was selected for its special appeal: its difficulty makes it a good benchmark. In the same way the Pac-Man problem is especially interesting as it captures the problem of survival in the abstract. The Pac-Man has to feed itself and survive in the face of predators. It has primitive sensors that can identify food and foes as well as motor capability. As such it is an excellent test bed to study whether GP can successfully find a good control strategy. Furthermore, the GP operations are so simple you can imagine how they might be done neurally in terms of changing wiring patterns introducing a changing control structure. Thus the evolutionary roots of the algorithm may be translatable into neural growth.

Tables 13.2 and 13.3 show the GP encoding of the problem. The two nonterminals appear as interior nodes of the tree and allow the Pac-Man to change behavior based on current conditions. The terminals either move the Pac-Man in the maze or take a measurement of the current environment, but they cannot call other functions.

Table 13.2 The GP Pac-Man nonterminals (control functions). (After Koza, 1992.)

Control Function Name	Purpose
If-Blue (IFB)	A two-argument branching operator that executes the first branch if the monsters are blue; otherwise the second.
If-Less-Than-or-Equal (IFLTE)	A four-argument branching operator that compares its second argument to its first. If it is less, the third argument is executed; otherwise the fourth is executed.

Table 13.3 The GP Pac-Man terminals. (After Koza, 1992.)

Terminal Function Name	Purpose
Advance-to-Pill (APILL)	Move toward nearest uneaten energizer
Retreat-from-Pill (RPILL)	Move away from nearest uneaten energizer
Distance-to-Pill (DPILL)	Distance to nearest uneaten energizer
Advance-to-Monster-A (AGA)	Move toward monster A
Retreat-from-Monster-A (RGA)	Move away from monster A
Distance-to-Monster-A (DISA)	Distance to monster A
Advance-to-Monster-B (AGB)	Move toward monster B
Retreat-from-Monster-B (RGB)	Move away from monster B
Distance-to-Monster-B (DISB)	Distance to monster B
Advance-to-Food (AFOOD)	Move toward nearest uneaten food
Distance-to-Food (DISD)	Distance to nearest food
Advance-to-Fruit (AFRUIT)	Move toward nearest fruit
Distance-to-Fruit (DISF)	Distance to nearest fruit

Figure 13.6 shows the solution obtained in a run of GP after 35 generations.[4] Note the form of the solution. The program solves the problem almost by rote, since the environment is similar each time. The monsters appear at the same time and move in the same way (more or less) each time. The regularities in the environment are incorporated directly into the program code. Thus while the solution is better than what a human programmer might come up with, it is very brittle and would not work well if the environment changed significantly.

The dynamics of GP can also be illustrated with this example. Figure 13.7 shows how the population evolves over time. Plotted are the number of individuals with a given fitness value as a function of both fitness value and generations. An obvious feature of the graph is that the maximum fitness value increases as a function of generations. However, an interesting subsidiary feature of the graph is the dynamics of genetic programming. Just as in the analysis of GAs, fit schemata will tend to

```
0 (IFB
1   (IFB
2    (IFLTE (AFRUIT)(AFRUIT)
3    (IFB
4      (IFB
5       (IFLTE
6        (IFLTE
          (AGA)
          (DISA)
7,8        (IFB (IFLTE
               (DISF)
               (AGA)
               (DPILL)
9              (IFLTE (DISU)(AGA)
                 (AGA)
10               (IFLTE (AFRUIT)(DISU)
                   (AFRUIT)
10,9,8             (DISA))))
8            (IFLTE (AFRUIT)(RGA)
               (IFB (DISA) 0)
8,7            (DISA)))
6          (DPILL))
         (IFB
7          (IFB (AGA)
8            (IFLTE
9              (IFLTE
                 (IFLTE (AFRUIT)(AFOOD)(DISA)(DISA))
                 (AFRUIT)
                 O
9                (IFB (AGA) 0))
               (DPILL)
               (IFLTE (AFRUIT)(DPILL)(RGA)(DISF))
8,7            (AFRUIT)))
           0)
         (AGA)
5       (RGA))
4     (AFRUIT))

3   (IFLTE
4     (IFLTE (RGA) (AFRUIT)(AFOOD)(AFOOD))
      (IFB(DPILL)(IFLTE (RGA)(APILL)(AFOOD)(DISU)))
5     (IFLTE
        (IFLTE (RGA)(AFRUIT)(AFOOD)(RPILL))
        (IFB (AGA) (DISB))
        (IFB (AFOOD) 2)
5       (IFB (DISB) (AFOOD)))
4,3     (IFB (DPILL) (AFOOD))))
2   (RPIL))
3   (IFB (DISB)
4     (IFLTE
        (DISU)
        0
        (AFOOD)
4,3,2   (AGA)))
2   (IFB (DISU)
3     (IFLTE
        (DISU)
        (DISU)
4       (IFLTE
5         (IFLTE (AFRUIT)
            (AFOOD)
            (DPILL)
5           (DISA))
          (AFRUIT)
          0
4         (IFB (AGA) 0))
3,2,1     (RGB))))
```

Figure 13.6 Program code that plays Pac-Man shows the ad hoc nature of the solution generated by GP. The numbers at the line beginnings indicate the level of indentation in the LISP code. (After Koza, 1992.)

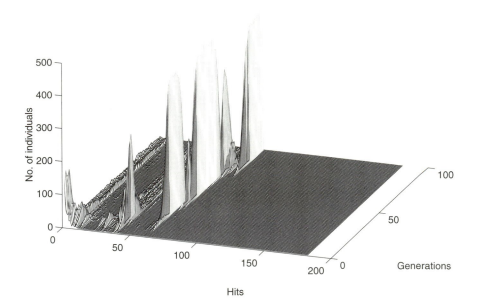

Figure 13.7 The dynamics of GP is illustrated by tracking the fitness of individuals as a function of generations. The vertical axis shows the number of individuals with a given fitness value. The horizontal axes show the fitness values and the generations. The peaks in the figure show clearly the effects of good discoveries. The fittest of the individuals rapidly saturate almost the whole population. (From Rosca and Ballard, 1996.)

increase in the population exponentially, and that fact is illustrated here. When a fit individual is discovered, the number of individuals with that fitness level rapidly increases until saturation. At the same time the sexual reproduction operators are working to make the population more diverse; that is, they are working to break up this schema and increase the diversity of the population. Once the number of this schema has saturated, then the diversifying effects of the sexual reproduction can catch up to the slowed growth rate of individuals with the new schema.

13.4 ANALYSIS

Since the performance of GP is too difficult to approach theoretically, we can attempt to characterize it experimentally.[5] The experimental approach is to observe the behavior of the algorithm on a variety of different runs of GP while varying N_G and N_p, and then attempt to draw some general conclusions. The most elementary parameter to measure is the probability of generating a solution at a particular generation k using a population size N_p. Call this $P_k(N_p)$, and let the cumulative probability of finding a solution up to and including generation i be given by

$$P(N_G, i) = \sum_{k=1}^{i} P_k(N_p)$$

One might think that P_k would increase monotonically with k so that using more generations would inevitably lead to a solution, but the experimental evidence shows otherwise. The fitness of individuals tends to plateau, meaning that the search for a solution has gotten stuck in a local minimum. Thus for most cases P_k eventually decreases with k. The recourse is to assume that successive experiments are independent and find the optimum with repeated runs that use different initial conditions.

A simple formula dictates the number of runs needed based on empirical success measures. This process leads to a trade-off between population size and multiple runs.

Assuming the runs are independent, you can estimate the number needed as long as $P(N_p, i)$ is known. This process works as follows. Let the probability of getting the answer after G generations be P_A. Then P_A is related to the number of experiments r by

$$P_A = 1 - [1 - P(N_p, G)]^r$$

Since the variable of interest is r, take logarithms of both sides,

$$\ln (1 - P_A) = r \ln [1 - P(N_p, G)]$$

or

$$r = \frac{\ln \varepsilon}{\ln [1 - P(N_p, G)]}$$

where ε is the error, $(1 - P_A)$.

These formulas allow you to get rough estimates on the GP algorithm for a particular problem, but a more basic question that you might have is about the efficacy of GP versus ordinary random search. Could one do as well by just taking the search effort and expending it by testing randomly generated examples? It turns out that the answer to this question is problem dependent, but for most hard problems the experimental evidence is that the performance of GP is much better than random search.[6]

13.5 MODULES

A striking feature of the Pac-Man solution shown in Figure 13.6 is its non-hierarchical structure. Each piece of the program is generated without taking advantage of similarities with other parts of the code. In the same way the parity problem would be a lot easier to solve if functions that solved subproblems could be used. Ideally one would like to define a hierarchy of functions, but it is not at all apparent how to do so. The obvious way would be to denote a subtree as a function and then add it to the library of functions that can be used in the GP algorithm. In LISP, the function call (FUNC X Y) would simply be replaced by a defined function name, say FN001, whose definition would be (FUNC X Y), and the rest of the computations would proceed as in the standard algorithm. The problem with this idea is the potential explosion in the number of functions. You cannot allow functions of all sizes in the GP algorithm owing to the expense of testing them. Each program is a tree containing subprograms as subtrees. Naively testing all subtrees in a population increases the workload by a factor of N^2. However, it is possible to test small trees that have terminals at their leaves efficiently by using a data structure that keeps track of them.[7] This way the price of testing the trees is reduced to a manageable size. Thus to make modules, all trees of size less than M are tested for some M that is chosen to be practical computationally.

The modular version of GP for the parity problem tests each of these small subtrees to see if they solve the problem for their subset of inputs. If they do, then each of those subtrees is made a function with the number of arguments equal to the variables used in the subtree. This function is then added to the pool of nonterminals and can be used anywhere in the population. This process is recursive. Once a new function is added to the nonterminal pool, it can be used as part of yet newer function compositions. If later generations solve a larger parity problem using the new function as a component, they can be treated in the same way: another new function is added to the nonterminal set. These constraints are formalized in Algorithm 13.2.

The modular approach works spectacularly well for parity, as shown in Table 13.4. Consider the entries for the 5 parity problem. Genetic programming without modules requires 50 generations, whereas the same problem can be solved in only 5 generations using modular GP. The reason, of course, is that functions that solve the parity of subsets of the data are enormously helpful as components of the larger solution.

Figure 13.8 shows the generation and use of new functions in the course of solving the 8 parity problem. In the course of the solution, functions that

Algorithm 13.2   Modular Genetic Programming

Choose a population size.

Choose the number of generations N_G.

Initialize the population.

Repeat the following for N_G generations:

1. Select a given number of pairs of individuals from the population probabilistically after assigning each structure a probability proportional to observed performance.

2. Copy the selected structure(s), then apply *operators* to them to produce new structure(s).

3. Select other elements at random and replace them with the new structure(s).

a. Test all the subtrees of size less than M. If there are any subtrees that solve a subproblem, add them to the nonterminal set.
b. Update the subtree data set.

4. Observe and record the fitness of the new structure.

Output the fittest individual as the answer.

Table 13.4 Comparison of GP and modular GP for parity problems of different sizes. Table entry is the generation at which the solution was found. Standard GP fails to find a solution to the even-8 parity problem after 50 generations, but modular GP solves the same problem at generation 10.

Method	Even-3	Even-4	Even-5	Even-8
GP	5	23	50	
Modular GP	2	3	5	10

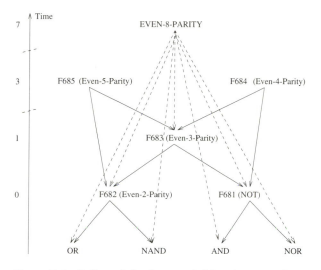

Figure 13.8 Call graph for the extended function set in the even-8 parity example showing the generation when each function was discovered. For example, even-5 parity was discovered at generation three and uses even-3 parity discovered at generation one and even-2 parity and NOT, each appearing at generation zero. (From Rosca and Ballard, 1994.)[8]

solved the 2, 3, 4, and 5 parity problem were generated at generations 0, 1, 3, and 7, respectively. The specific code for each of these functions is shown in Table 13.5. These functions may look cumbersome, but they are readily interpretable. Function F681 is the negation of a function of a single argument. Note that this was not in the initial function library. Function F682 computes the parity of its two arguments. Not surprisingly, this function is extremely useful in larger parity problems, and you can see that it is used extensively in the final solution shown in the table.

13.5.1 Testing for a Module Function

The previous strategy for selecting modules used all the trees less than some height bound. This strategy can be improved by keeping track of *differential fitness*. The idea is that promising modules will confer a fitness on their host that is greater than the average, that is,

$$\Delta f_s = f_{host} - f_{parents}$$

Table 13.5 Important steps in the evolutionary trace for a run of even-8 parity. "LAMBDA" is a generic construct used to define the body of new functions. (From Rosca and Ballard, 1994.)[9]

Generation 0. New functions
[F681]: (LAMBDA (D3) (NOR D3 (AND D3 D3)));
[F682]: (LAMBDA (D4 D3) (NAND (OR D3 D4) (NAND D3 D4)))

Generation 1. New function
[F683]: (LAMBDA (D4 D5 D7) (F682 (F681 D4) (F682 D7 D5)))

Generation 3. New functions
[F684]: (LAMBDA (D4 D5 D0 D1 D6) (F683 (F683 D0 D6 D1) (F681 D4)
(OR D5 D5)));
[F685]: (LAMBDA (D1 D7 D6 D5) (F683 (F681 D1) (AND D7 D7) (F682 D5 D6)))

Generation 7. The solution found is: (OR (F682 (F682 (F683 D4 D2 D6) (NAND (NAND (AND D6 D1) (F681 D5)) D1)) (F682 (F683 D5 D0 D3) (NOR D7 D2))) D5)

Thus a more useful measure of subroutine fitness is to select candidates that have a positive differential fitness. With this modification, you can use Algorithm 13.3 to select subroutines.

13.5.2   When to Diversify

The distribution of the fitness among individuals in a population is captured by the fitness histogram, which plots, for a set of discrete fitness ranges, the number of individuals within each range. Insight into the dynamics of propagation of individuals using subroutines can be seen by graphing the fitness histogram as a function of generation, as is done in Figure 13.9. This figure shows that once a good individual appears it grows exponentially to saturate the population. These individuals are subsequently replaced by an exponential growth of a fitter individual. The stunning improvement is seen for the example of Pac-Man. Comparing this result with that of Figure 13.7, the plot of the fitness histogram shows that not only is the population more diversified, but also that the fitness increases faster and ultimately settles at a larger point.

Algorithm 13.3   Selecting a Subroutine

1. Select a set of promising individuals that have positive differential fitness.

2. Compute the number of activations of each such individual.

3. Select all blocks of small height and high activation.

4. For each block b with terminals T_s do the following:

a. Create a new subroutine having a random subset of the terminals T_s with body (b, T_s).

b. Choose a program that uses the block b, and replace it with the new subroutine.

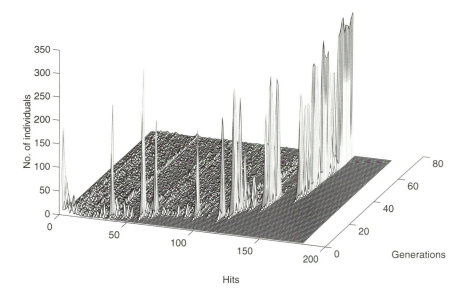

Figure 13.9 The dynamics of GP with subroutines is illustrated by tracking the fitness of individuals as a function of generations. The vertical axis shows the number of individuals with a given fitness value. The horizontal axes show the fitness values and the generations. The beneficial effects of subroutines can be seen by comparing this figure with Figure 13.7. (From Rosca and Ballard, 1996.)

Further insight into the efficacy of the modular algorithm can be obtained by studying the entropy of the population. Let us define an entropy measure by equating all individuals with the same fitness measure. If fitness is normalized, then it can be used like a probability. Then entropy is just

$$E = \sum f_i \log f_i$$

When the solution is not found, as in nonlocal GP, the search process decreases the diversity of the population, as shown by the top graph in Figure 13.10. This result is symptomatic of getting stuck in a local fitness maximum. But the nonlocal search of modular GP continually introduces diversity into the population. This process in turn keeps the entropy measure high, as shown in the lower graph in Figure 13.10. This behavior can be used to detect when a solution is stuck. If the entropy is decreasing but the fitness is constant, then it is extremely likely that the population is being dominated by a few types of individuals of maximum fitness. In this case the diversity of the population can be increased by increasing the rate of adding new modules.

Finally, you can see the effects of the subroutine strategy from Table 13.6, which compares runs from GP with and without subroutines.

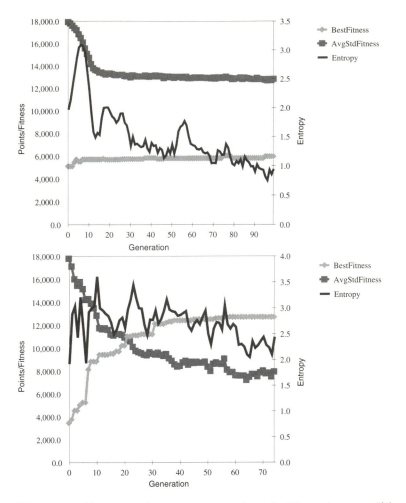

Figure 13.10 Entropy used as a measure to evaluate the GP search process. If the solution is found or if the population is stuck on a local fitness maximum, the entropy of the population tends to slowly decrease (*top*). In searching for a solution the diversity of a population typically increases, as reflected in the fluctuations in entropy in the modular case (*bottom*). (From Rosca and Ballard, 1996.)

Table 13.6 Comparison between solutions obtained with standard GP, subroutines, and a carefully hand-designed program. The GP parameters have the following values: population size = 500; crossover rate = 90%; reproduction rate = 10% (no mutation). During evolution, fitness is determined by simulation in 1 or 3 different environments. Each table entry shows the total number of points of an evolved Pac-Man controller for the corresponding GP implementation and, in parentheses, the generation when that solution was discovered. For all entries, the best results over 100 simulations were taken.

GP		Subroutines		Hand
1	3	1	3	
6380 (67)	4293 (17)	9840 (20)	5793 (36)	5630

13.6 SUMMARY

The features of GP search are qualitatively similar to that of GAs. Once an individual of slightly increased differential fitness is produced, its features tend to spread exponentially through the population. During this period the mechanism of sexual reproduction helps this process along. However, once the features saturate the population, sexual reproduction continues by breaking up program segments in the course of searching for new above-average features. Since most changes tend to be harmful, the course of sexual reproduction and schemata growth can be seen as being in dynamic balance.

In the world, nature provides the fitness function. This function is extremely complicated, reflecting the complexity of the organism in its milieu. Inside the GP algorithm, however, fitness must be estimated, using both *a priori* knowledge and knowledge from the search process itself. The power of subroutines in this context is that they provide a way of pooling the results of the organism's experiments across the population. Thus they provide a way of estimating the effects of a schema en route to a solution.

NOTES

1. John R. Koza, *Genetic Programming: On the Programming of Computers by Means of Natural Selection* (Cambridge, MA: MIT Press, Bradford, 1992).

2. Actually, one does not put all the integers into the terminal set. Instead a function *random-integer* is used; whenever it is called, a random integer is generated and inserted into the program.

3. The Pac-Man example was introduced by Koza in *Genetic Programming* and refined by Justinian P. Rosca and Dana H. Ballard in "Discovery of Subroutines in Genetic Programming," Chapter 9 in P. Angeline and K. E. Kinnear, Jr., eds., *Advances in Genetic Programming 2* (Cambridge, MA: MIT Press, 1996).

4. Koza, *Genetic Programming*.

5. This analysis was first done by Koza in *Genetic Programming*.

6. See, for example, Chapter 9 of Koza, *Genetic Programming*.

7. Justinian P. Rosca and Dana H. Ballard, "Genetic Programming with Adaptive Representations," TR 489, Computer Science Department, University of Rochester, February 1994.

8. Justinian P. Rosca and Dana H. Ballard, "Hierarchical Self-Organization in Genetic Programming," in W. W. Cohen and H. Hirsch, eds., *Machine Learning: Proceedings of the 11th International Conference* (San Francisco: Morgan Kaufmann Publishers, Inc.: 1994), p. 255.

9. Ibid.

EXERCISES

1. Try to come up with a simpler set of actions for the Pac-Man problem that reapplies the program after each step.

2. Verify the relationship between population size and cumulative success rate using the parity problem.

3. Implement a solution to the Pac-Man problem that uses modules.

4. Using the solution to the previous problem, add code to test for the portion of the code in individuals that is unused.

5. Compare the size of a program—as measured by using subroutines as primitives—to the equivalent solution cast in terms of the original primitive set.

6. Assuming changes are random and trees are balanced, derive a formula for the probability $P(d)$ that the change made to a tree occurs at depth d.

7. Simulate the 5-parity problem with GP and GP-with-subroutines.

8. Compare the solution for the preceding problem to the time taken to generate random trees.

14 Summary

An animal that depends on its brain for survival benefits from having a large repertoire of behavioral programs that can execute quickly. For primates, however, brain size is limited by what is practical to push through the birth canal, and program speed is limited by the speed of the neuron. Thus there is enormous pressure for the development of good algorithms. Such algorithms can be rated by a minimum-description-length (MDL) principle, which balances the work that the algorithms do against their own internal cost. This has the effect of accounting for both the speed and size of the program.

Complex systems are very difficult to analyze. For there to be any hope at all they almost have to be organized hierarchically. The brain exhibits extensive hierarchical structures in both space and time. The algorithms in this book are similarly organized.

14.1 LEARNING TO REACT: MEMORIES

The fastest way to compute is by storing what to do in different situations in memories, or "look-up tables." A stimulus pattern is sensed, and a response can be generated as fast as the answer can be looked up using neural circuitry. Content-addressable memory (CAM) is one way of learning the patterns such that the patterns can be highly noise-tolerant. That is, a CAM can fill in the missing parts of a memory appropriately even when it is distorted and has missing parts. If the CAM is limited to neurons that just represent the initial sensory data, its categorization is limited. The addition of neurons that are not directly connected to the input data, "hidden units," allows the system to recognize dissimilar sensory patterns as instances of the same situation, and vice versa. The algorithms for using additional units were initially supervised with an externally provided signal, but newer developments allow supervisory signals to be derived from the data themselves. It is likely that the cortex and cerebellum are CAMs.

At the moment there is not a unified theory on the design of the brain's CAM, and different models emphasize different memory features. Kalman filtering, based on the MDL principle and discussed in Chapter 7, emphasizes the need to predict the input quickly. Independent components, discussed in Chapter 9 and based on an entropy measure, emphasizes the need to factor the input.

14.2   LEARNING DURING A LIFETIME: PROGRAMS

Programs compose look-up table operations to form larger behaviors. Such programs can be thought of as using the CAM by specifying sequences of memories.

At the more abstract level of a program, the problem is to define both a problem state space and operators that express the transitions between different states. It is likely that the entire brain is involved in this process, but that the most central structures are located in the basal ganglia.

An extremely useful way of modeling programs that handles uncertainty is to define internal or "hidden" states using only local context and to allow probabilistic transitions between states. Such a system is called a *hidden Markov model*. Such a local view may be the only thing that is practical to compute.

Hidden Markov models (HMMs) provide the necessary substrate for describing the fundamental mechanism of writing the brain's programs: secondary reward. Actual rewards in the world are in the future. To take an action in the present, the brain's programs must have a way of estimating these rewards. Reinforcement learning may be the most plausible way for the brain to make such estimates. It associates rewards with transitions in HMMs such that paths through the HMM tend to maximize reward. Reinforcement learning systems have recently been extended so that they can learn state spaces and operators in modest problem sizes, as described in Chapter 11. What they cannot do yet, but need to do, is incorporate mechanisms for simulating the program in the absence of input. Such simulations are ubiquitous in the brain, as they allow it to try out situations of uncertain reward mentally without risking its physical self.

14.3   LEARNING ACROSS GENERATIONS: SYSTEMS

Look-up tables and reinforcement strategies can reconfigure the existing structures, but cannot alter the hardware design. For that purpose, genetic changes are needed. Genetic algorithms model the alteration of the genes during reproduction in order to create new architectural forms. These algorithms can be understood as experimenting with brain hardware. Changing hardware is a slow process that operates across millions of generations, but it still can be modeled as an algorithmic process.

Genetic algorithms use strings of symbols to represent the genetic code and a fitness function to score the code. Populations of strings represent a species, and the most fit species represents the best solution found so far. The operations of sexual combination are translated into operations on the symbol strings, so that the population of symbol strings can evolve through "sexual" reproduction. Search proceeds by preferentially selecting the fittest strings for reproduction. What this search mechanism provides is a way of selecting fit structures without a *deus ex machina*. Such structures propagate among the population just by virtue of having conferred fitness on their hosts. We might speculate on how something like the MDL principle was ever guessed, but once it is guessed it is easy to see how it becomes a standard feature of the population.

A more recent development is to represent individuals as actual programs. The genetic operations are carried out on the actual program code, and as a result, an individual is a functioning program. This procedure gives the fitness function less to do, as the program can be directly tested in the environment. In the real world the fitness function is provided. In the model world the fitness function must be guessed by the algorithm designer. Having individuals represented as programs with hierarchical internal structure allows the fitness function to be guessed by tracking the success of schemata among populations, as described in Chapter 13.

14.4 THE GRAND CHALLENGE REVISITED

Progress on computational models of the brain is so recent and is moving so swiftly that it is difficult to keep track of all the developments and the scientists who have furthered this enterprise. But certainly most would acknowledge the central role of David Marr, who formulated human vision in computational terms. Although Marr himself thought that neural models might be too detailed and thus obscure essential algorithmic features, his focus on the algorithmic approach was liberating, and the publication of his book in 1982 has been followed by the rapid growth of neural algorithms. These algorithms break with so many of the tenets of classical computing that the term *natural computation* has been used to describe them. Hopefully you have been persuaded at this point that understanding such computation is indeed central to understanding the brain and that progress is being made in answering Richards' central question:

Biological systems have available through their senses only very limited information about the external world. . . . How can an incomplete description, encoded within neural states, be sufficient to direct the survival and successful adaptive behavior of a living system?[1]

NOTE

1. Whitman Richards, ed., *Natural Computation* (Cambridge, MA: MIT Press, 1988).

Index

Hypercube, content-addressable memory
(CAM), 147
Hyperplanes, perceptrons, 165

Identity matrix, linear algebra, 91–92
Image coding, minimum description length
(MDL), 47–48
Independent component analysis,
unsupervised learning, 201–3
Information theory
classification, 44–46
content and channel capacity, 38–39
entropy, 39–41
fitness function, 31–32, 37–44
reversible codes, 41–44
Initial state, heuristic search, 60
Insect behavior, program data model, 27–29
Instability, nonlinear dynamic systems,
106–7
Instance, tree data structures, 250
Inverse matrix, linear algebra, 91
Inversion operators
genetic algorithms, 265
LISP genetic programming, 279
Irreversible codes, information theory, 43–44

Jacobian matrices, dynamic systems, 97–98

k-armed bandit problem, one-step
Q-learning algorithm, 236
Kalman filtering, 159–60, 295–96
Kanerva memories
applications, 151–58
defined, 144
implementation, 153–55
performance criteria, 155–57
Kohonen learning
defined, 186
natural topologies, 191–94
neural network memory models, 141
topological constraints, 190–91
traveling salesman problem, 191
Kolmogorov, A. N., 11

Labeling, neural network memory models,
140
Lagrange multipliers
closest point to a circle example, 119
optimal control, 121–30
optimization theory, 113, 114–15, 118–20
Laplace transform methods, optimal
control, 125–26
Layered feedforward network, neural
network memory models, 140

Learning. *See also* Competitive learning;
Supervised learning; Unsupervised
learning
architectures of, 20–21
behavioral programs, 207–12
lifetime learning, 20
natural computation, 9–10, 14–15
Learning algorithms, 14–15, 18–21
Learning by watching (LBW),
reinforcement learning, 230–31, 241–42
Learning models, program modeling, 211
Learning with an external critic (LEC),
reinforcement learning, 230–31, 241–42
Likelihood ratio, information classification,
44–46
Linear algebra, data management, 88–91
Linear differential equations (LDE),
dynamic systems, 101–3
Linear independence, data and coordinate
systems, 73–75
Linear space
data compression, 71–72
Markov decision process (MDP), 243–44
Linear systems
dynamics, 27, 98–104
eigenvalues and eigenvectors, 103–4
optimal control, noise and, 126–27
radioactive decay, 99
system dynamics, 95–96
undamped harmonic oscillator, 99–101
Linear transformations, linear algebra, 90
LISP programming language, genetic
programming, 277–80
Local minima
in Hopfield memory, 150–51
optimization theory, 115–16, 131n.2
single-layered networks, 117–18
Logic, biological state spaces, 68n.3
Loss function
optimal control, 121
optimization theory, 114
Lyapunov function
Hopfield memory, 149–51
nonlinear systems, 106, 108–9

Marginal stability, nonlinear dynamic
systems, 106–7
Markers, Markov decision process (MDP),
244–46
Markov decision process (MDP)
bad state avoidance, 244–46
maze problem, 232–33
pole balancing, 233
reinforcement learning, 229–33

Euler-Lagrange method, 121–27
  optimization theory, 114, 121–30
Optimization theory
  dynamic programming, 127–30
  Euler-Lagrange method, 121–27
  Lagrange multipliers, 118–20
  minimization algorithms, 115–18
  minimum description length (MDL)
    and, 11
  natural computation and, 19–20, 113–30
Orthogonality, data and coordinate
  systems, 73–75
Othello game, 65–66

Pac-Man example
  genetic programming, 282–92
  program coding, 284–85
Parameter maximization, hidden Markov
  models, 222
Parasite coevolution, genetic algorithms,
  271–73
Parity problems
  genetic programming, 281–82
  modular genetic programming, 288–90
Partial derivatives
  dynamic systems, 97
  single-layered networks, 118
Partially observable Markov decision
  process (MDP), 231, 243–52
Pattern discrimination
  multimodal data, 197–201
  partial pattern completion, hierarchical
    memory, 138
Penrose, Roger, 2
Perceptrons
  defined, 164
  learning rule, 165–67, 181n.2
  supervised learning and, 164–67
Perceptual aliases
  Markov decision process (MDP), 243–46
  temporal sequences, 247–48
Phenotype
  evolutionary learning, 257
  genetic algorithms, 272–73
Plys, two-person games, 64
Poisson distribution, 34–35
  Kanerva memory, 156
Pole balancing, Markov decision process,
  233
Policy improvement theorem,
  reinforcement learning, 230, 234–35
Polynomial complexity, computational
  theory and, 9
Positive matrices, eigenvalues of, 78–79

Probability density function, 35–37
  information classification, 44–45
  random vectors, 80–84
Probability distributions
  continuous distributions, 35–37
  discrete distributions, 33–35
  fitness function, 33–38
Probability of observation sequence, hidden
  Markov models, 222–24
Probability theory
  Bayes' rule, 31–33
  laws of, 48–50
Probability vector, Markov models, 216
Programs for learning behavior, 19, 27,
  55–67, 207, 296
  brain subsystems using chemical
    rewards, 207–9
  learning models, 211–12
  rewards, 210–11
  system integration, 211
Proportionality, information capacity,
  38–39
Prototype points, unsupervised learning,
  185–86
Provisional backed-up value (PBV), alpha
  and beta cutoffs, 66

Q-function (action-value function)
  Q-learning, 235–36
  reinforcement learning, 234–35
Q-learning algorithm, 230, 235–36
  tree data structures, 250–51
Quadratic equations, minimization
  algorithms, 117
Quantum physics, computational models
  and, 2

Racing for fitness problem, genetic
  algorithms, 270–71
Radial basis functions, content-addressable
  memory (CAM), 159
Radioactive decay, linear systems, 99
Random walking, temporal difference
  learning, 242–43
Real-valued random variables, probability
  density function, 35–36
Recurrent networks
  defined, 164
  perceptrons, 164–67
  supervised learning applications, 174–78
Redundancy
  information theory, 38
  unsupervised learning, 185–86
Regular chains, Markov models, 217–18